A PRACTICAL ENGLISH—CHINESE LIBRARY OF TRADITIONAL CHINESE MEDICINE

PUBLISHING HOUSE OF SHANGHAI UNIVERSITY OF TRADITIONAL CHINESE MEDICINE

EDITOR—IN—CHIEF ZHANG ENQIN

BASIC THEORY OF TRADITIONAL CHINESE MEDICINE (II)

Written   by   Shi Lanhua
                  Zhang Enqin
                  Wang Min
Translated by   Hu Zhaoyun
                  Han Yufang
Revised   by   Zhang Qingling
                  Zhang Enqin

英汉对照
实用中医文库

主　编　张恩勤

中医基础理论

●下册

编著　史兰华　张恩勤
　　　　王　敏

翻译　胡兆云　韩毓昉

审校　张庆龄　张恩勤

上海中医药大学出版社

THE GUIDING COMMITTEE
OF THE LIBRARY

Director Hu Ximing
Deputy Directors Wang Lei Yan Shiyun
Members (in the order of the number of Chinese strokes in the surnames)

Wan Deguang	Wang Yongyan	Lu Chengzhi	Lü Tongjie
Sun Guojie	Liu Chonggang	Liu Mingde	Li Keshao
Su Shisheng	Zhang Zhiyuan	Zhang Canjia	Zhang Minghe
Zhang Qiwen	Zhang Zhenyu	Chen Keji	Chen Weiyang
Zou Ling	Qiu Maoliang	Qiu Dewen	Zhou Fengwu
Zhou Zhongying	Zhou Ciqing	Shang Zhichang	Xiang Ping
Xu Guoqian	Gao Chuantang	Cui Mingxiu	Huang Wenxing
Huang Xiaokai	Huang Jiade		

CHIEF AUTHORS OF THE LIBRARY

Advisors   Dong Jianhua Liu Duzhou Deng Tietao
Editor-in-Chief Zhang Enqin
Associate Editors-in-Chief of TCM (in the order of the number of Chinese strokes in the surnames)

Shi Lanhua	Zhang Wengao	Zhang Zhigang	Zhang Jidong
Li Dunqing	Zhao Chunxiu	Dang Yi	Wei Jiwu

Associate Editors-in-Chief of English (in the order of the number of Chinese strokes in the surnames)

Yu Wenping	Wang Zhikui	Li Yulin	Li Yanfu
Xiao Gong	Zhang Minglun	Hou Mingjun	Wen Hongrui

THE EDITING AND TRANSLATING
COMMITTEE OF THE LIBRARY

Director Zou Jilong

Deputy Directors (in the order of the number of Chinese strokes in the surnames)

Tian Daihua	Cong Laiting	Sun Xigang	Wu Guanghua
Chen Guangzhen	Jing Jie	Gao Heting	Cao Yixun
Cheng Yichun	Cai Jianqian		

Members (in the order of the number of Chinese strokes in the surnames)

Yu Shufang	Wang Jun	Wang Min	Wang Qi
Wang Chenying	Wang Baoxiang	Wang Guocai	Wang Ziwei
Yin Hongan	Tai Shuren	Mao Chun	Zuo Lianjun
Shi Renhua	Mi Li	Bi Yongsheng	Chi Yongli
Bao Xianmin	Lü Jianping	Qu Jingfeng	Zhu Xiaoming
Qiao Mingqi	Sun Hua	Sun Xiao	Sun Guangren
Sun Hengshan	Liu Wenjing	Liu Zhongyuan	Liu Rongyuan
Liu Jiayi	Liu Peilu	Jiang Xiuzheng	Mu Junzheng
Shi Xiuqin	Yang Min	Li Yan	Li Wei
Li Changsheng	Li Xuezhen	Li Shaoqing	Li Qingxiu
Zhang Shaohua	Zhang Yuxi	Zhang Qingling	Zhang Zhongtian
Zhang Xuezeng	Zhang Shengxin	Jin Ruhua	Zheng Yi
Zheng Yanchen	Zheng Shouzeng	Zhao Shili	Zhao Laixi
Zhao Lanfeng	Hu Zhaoyun	Jiang Longsheng	Jiang Xueting
Jiang Jingxian	Shao Guanyong	Gao Yan	Gao Yi
Gao Hongren	Gao Yongli	Nie Qingxi	Xia Yunbin
Shang Zhenyong	Liang Shuqun	Yan Ping	Cui Hongjiang
Cui Jipin	Cao Zhiqun	Dong Xinhua	Dong Xuemei
Han Yan	Han Yufang	Xie Guangfa	

Director of the Committee Office Tai Shuren

《英汉对照实用中医文库》编译委员会

主 任 邹积隆

副主任 （以姓氏笔划为序）

田代华　丛莱庭　孙希刚　吴光华　陈广祯
经　捷　高鹤亭　曹贻训　程益春　蔡剑前

委 员 （以姓氏笔划为序）

于淑芳　王　军　王　敏　王　琦　王陈应
王宝祥　王国才　王紫薇　尹洪安　太树人
毛　淳　左连君　史仁华　米　鹏　毕永升
迟永利　包献民　吕建平　曲京峰　朱晓明
乔明琦　孙　华　孙　校　孙广仁　孙衡山
刘文敬　刘仲源　刘荣源　刘家义　刘培禄
江秀贞　牟俊贞　时秀芹　杨　敏　李　延
李　巍　李长生　李学珍　李绍卿　李清修
张少华　张玉玺　张庆龄　张忠田　张学增
张盛心　金汝华　郑　艺　郑延辰　郑守曾
赵世立　赵来玺　赵岚峰　胡兆云　姜龙盛
姜学亭　姜静娴　邵冠勇　高　艳　高　教
高洪仁　皋永利　聂庆喜　夏运斌　商振勇
梁舒群　阎　平　崔洪江　崔继聘　曹志群
董新华　董雪梅　韩　燕　韩毓昉　解广法

办公室主任 太树人

Preface

The books in series, entitled *"A Practical English-Chinese Library of Traditional Chinese Medicine"*, are edited with a view to disseminating the theory and knowledge of traditional Chinese medicine (TCM) across the world, promoting academic exchanges on medical science between China and other countries, and meeting with the ever-increasing international interest in TCM, so as to make it serve the interests of all nations and benefit entire mankind. This library is the first of its kind in China.

The library is composed of 12 books: *Basic Theory of TCM* (in two volumes), *Diagnostics of TCM, The Chinese Materia Medica, Prescriptions of TCM, Clinic of TCM* (in two volumes), *Health Preservation and Rehabilitation, Chinese Acupuncture and Moxibustion, Chinese Medicated Diet* and *Chinese Qigong*. The two other English-Chinese books —— *Rare Chinese Materia Medica* and *Highly Efficacious Chinese Patent Medicine* —— chiefly edited by me are also published simultaneously along with this library.

The authors and editors of the series strive to abide by the following principles: maintaining the systematism, integrity, practicability and adaptability in terms of TCM theory; paying full attention to the organic connection between basic theory and clinical treatment, taking in the available results of scientific researches carried out at home and abroad in the

1

field of TCM; and being concise, precise, and easy to understand in the Chinese version, and correct and fluent in the English one. Some of the books mentioned above contain figures and coloured photos. It is our sincere hope that the books will turn out to be good teachers and reliable friends of those abroad who have begun to learn and practise TCM and Chinese, and provide help for those at home who wish to study TCM documents in English.

The component books of this library are written, translated, and edited through joint efforts of professors, associate professors, lecturers and medical research workers from Shandong TCM College and its affiliated hospital, Shandong Medical University and its affiliated hospital, Shandong University, Shandong Teachers Training University, Shandong Medical Academy, Shandong Provincial Anti-epidemic Station, China Academy of TCM, Nanjing TCM College, Shanghai TCM College, Beijing TCM College, etc.

In order to ensure that the present library is of good quality, we have sent its Chinese version for revision to Professor Zhou Fengwu, Professor Li Keshao who was once my tutor when I was a postgraduate student, Professor Xu Guoqian and Professor Zhang Zhenyu at Shandong TCM College, Professor Qiu Maoliang at Nanjing TCM College, and Professor Lu Tongjie, director of the Affiliated Hospital of Shandong TCM College; and the English version for proofreading to Professor Huang Xiaokai of Beijing Medical University, Professor Lu Chengzhi, head of the Foreign Languages Department of Shandong Medical University, Professor Huang Jiade of Shandong University, Mr. Huang Wenxing, professor of

2

pharmacology, Mme. Zou Ling, professor of gynecology and obstetrics, both working in Shandong Medical University, and our foreign friends, Ms. Beth Hocks, Australian teacher of English, Mr. Howard G. Adams, American teacher of English, and some others working in Jinan.

I am deeply indebted to Mr. Li Dichen, Editor-in-Chief of Publishing House of Shanghai TCM College, and his colleagues, Mme. Xu Ping, director of the Editorial Depatmrent, and Mr. Yao Yong, responsible editor, for their advice about drawing up an outline for compiling the library to ensure a success of it; to Mr. Chen Keji, professor of China Academy of TCM and advisor on traditional medicine to WHO, Professor Zhang Zhiyuan and Associate Professor Shao Guanyong of Shandong TCM College, Mr. Liu Chonggang, deputy head of the Yellow River Publishing House, for their valuable, instructive suggestions; and to responsible members at various levels, such as Mr. Hu Ximing, Chairman of the World Acupuncture and Moxibustion Association, vice-minister of the Ministry of public Health and chief of the Administrative Bureau of TCM and Pharmacy of the People's Republic of China, Mr. Zou Jilong, president of Shandong TCM College, Mr. Yan Shiyun, vice-president of Shanghai TCM College, Mr. Gao Heting, president of Beijing TCM College, Mr. Xiang Ping, vice president of Nanjing TCM College, and Mr. Shang Zhichang, president of Henan TCM College for their warm encouragement and indispensable support as well as their personal participation in compiling and checking the books.

TCM, which dates back to ancient times, has a unique

and profound theoretical system. The greater part of its terminology has particular denotations, and is matter-of-factly difficult to understand and translate. Inaccuracies in the library, therefore, are unavoidable. I hope that my friends in the TCM circle will oblige me with timely corrections.

May TCM spread all over the world and everyone under the heaven enjoy a long happy life.

May 20th, 1988 Dr. Zhang Enqin
Editor-in-Chief of *A Practical English-Chinese Library of Traditional Chinese Medicine,* Director of the Advanced Studies Department of Shandong TCM College

前　言

　　为扩大中医学在国际上的影响，促进中外医学学术交流，适应国外日趋发展的"中医热"形势，使传统的中医学走向世界，造福人类，我们编写了这套《英汉对照实用中医文库》。在国内，这尚属首部。

　　该文库包括《中医基础理论》（上、下册）、《中医诊断学》、《中药学》、《方剂学》、《中医临床各科》（上、下册）、《中医养生康复学》、《中国针灸》、《中国推拿》、《中国药膳》和《中国气功》，共十二个分册。与《文库》同时出版的还有其配套书——英汉对照《中国名贵药材》和《中国名优中成药》。

　　《英汉对照实用中医文库》的编译宗旨是：在理论上，努力保持中医学体系的系统性、完整性，突出实用性和针对性；在内容上，充分注意基础理论与临床治疗的有机联系，汲取国内外已公布的科研成果，以反映当代中医学术水平；在文字上，力求中文简明扼要，通俗易懂，译文准确流畅，并配有图表、彩照。我们竭诚希望《英汉对照实用中医文库》能成为国外读者学习中医、汉语的良师益友，同时也为国内读者学习中医专业英语提供帮助。

　　负责文库编写、翻译和审校的主要是山东中医学院及其附属医院、山东医科大学及其附属医院、山东大学、山东师范大学、山东省医学科学院、山东省卫生防疫站、中国中医研究院、南京中医学院，上海中医学院和北京中医学院等单位的部分教授、副教授、讲师和科研人员。

　　为确保文库质量，各分册中文稿还先后承蒙山东中医学院周凤梧教授、李克绍教授、徐国仟教授、张珍玉教授，南京中医学院邱茂良教授，山东中医学院附属医院院长吕同杰教授等审阅；英文稿先后承蒙北京医科大学英语教研室黄孝楷教授，山东医科大学英语教研室主任卢承志教授，山东大学外文系黄嘉德教授，山东医科大学药理教研室黄文兴教授、妇产科教研室邹玲教授以及澳大利亚籍教师 Beth Hocks 女士和美籍教师 Howard G. Adams 先生等审阅。

上海中医学院出版社总编辑李迪臣、编辑部主任徐平和责任编辑姚勇，亲自帮助我们修订编写大纲，指导编译工作；世界卫生组织传统医学顾问、中国中医研究院陈可冀教授，山东中医学院张志远教授、邵冠勇副教授，黄河出版社副社长刘崇刚，也为本文库的编译工作提出了许多宝贵的指导性意见；编译工作还得到了各级领导的支持和帮助，世界针灸学会联合会主席、中华人民共和国卫生部副部长兼国家中医药管理局局长胡熙明先生，山东中医学院院长邹积隆先生，上海中医学院副院长严世芸先生，北京中医学院院长高鹤亭先生，南京中医学院副院长项平先生和河南中医学院院长尚炽昌先生等，亲自参加编审并给予指导，在此一并表示衷心感谢！

由于中医学源远流长，其理论体系独特，不少名词术语深奥难解，译成英文，难度较大。故书中错误、欠妥之处在所难免，敬希国内外同道指正。

愿中医流传世界，求普天下人健康长寿。

主编　张恩勤

1988年5月20日

CONTENTS

目　　录

Basic Theory of Traditional Chinese

Medicine (II)

中医基础理论(下册)

Chapter One

PATHOGENIC FACTORS

What are pathogenic factors ? Pathogenic factors refer to the various kinds of factors that cause diseases, mainly including six exogenous factors, epidemic pathogenic factors, internal injury by seven emotions, improper diet, maladjustment of work and rest, and surgical trauma.

In recognizing pathogenic factors, besides understanding the objective conditions which may be pathogenic factors, traditional Chinese medicine is mainly based on the clinical manifestations of diseases, and inquires into the pathogenic factors through analyzing the symptoms and signs of diseases, thus providing a basis for treatment and medication. This method is called "determination of pathogenic factors based on the differentiation of symptoms and signs".

The classification of pathogenic factors varies among doctors of different times. For instance, *The Yellow Emperor's Canon of Internal Medicine* (722–221 B.C.) classifies them, for the first time, into two categories: *yin* and *yang*. Up to the Eastern Han Dynasty (25–220 A.D.), Zhang Zhongjing pointed out in his *Synopsis of the Golden Chamber* (219 A.D.) that the pathogenic factors of diseases could be classified into three categories. He said: "Though there are various kinds of diseases, they can not go beyond three categories: in the first category, pathogenic factors affect the channels and collaterals which further involve the viscera to cause internal diseases; in the second category, the four limbs and nine orifices are affected by way of blood vessels with pathological changes transmitted to each other resulting in blocked passage: diseases so

第 一 章

病 因

什么是病因？病因是指导致疾病发生的各种原因，主要有六淫、疠气、七情内伤、饮食不节、劳逸失度以及外伤等。

中医认识病因，除了解可能作为致病因素的客观条件外，主要是以病证的临床表现为依据，通过分析疾病的症状、体征来推求病因，为治疗用药提供依据，这种方法称为"辨证求因"。

关于病因的分类，历代医家各不相同。如《内经》首次将其分为阴阳两类。至东汉，张仲景在《金匮要略》中指出，疾病发生有三条途径，即所谓："千般疢难，不越三条：一者，经络受邪入脏腑，为内所因也；二者，四肢九窍，血脉相传，壅塞不通，为外皮肤所中也；三者，房室、金刃、虫兽所伤。以此详之，病由都

formed are through the external skin; the third category includes diseases caused by intemperance in sexual life, incised wounds and bites and stings by animals and insects. Under the three categories, the causes of all diseases can be covered without exception." From "though there are various kinds of diseases, they can not go beyond three categories" in *Synopsis of the Golden Chamber*, Chen Wuze of the Song Dynasty (960–1279) put forward the "Triple-Etiology Doctrine" which classifies three categories of pathogenic factors, i.e. external invasions by six exogenous factors are exopathic factors; internal injury by the emotional upset are endopathic factors; improper diet as well as traumatic injuries including injuries from falls, fractures, contusion and sprain, incised wounds and injuries by insects and animals are non-endo-exopathic factors. I think that various pathogenic factors are all exopathic factors, whereas the relative asthenia of the vital-*qi* of the human body is the endopathic factor. Under general circumstances, exopathic factors become operative through endopathic factors. Now a few common pathogenic factors are dealt with respectively as follows:

Section 1

Six Exogenous Factors

Six exogenous factors is a general term for the six climatic conditions in excess as pathogenic factors: wind, cold, summerheat, dampness, dryness and fire. In normal condition, they are actually six normal climatic variations of nature, and are therefore also called "six natural factors". Human beings live in nature and have a certain adaptability to various climatic variations, so the six normal natural factors can not make people contract diseases. But if the climatic variations are too unusual,

尽。"宋代陈无择又引申《金匮要略》"千般疢难，不越三条"之意，

提出了"三因学说"，即六淫外袭为外因，情志内伤为内因，饮食饥

饱以及跌仆、金刃、虫兽所伤为不内外因。笔者认为，各种致病

因素均属外因，而人体正气的相对虚弱才是内因。在一般情况下，

外因是通过内因而起作用的。现将几种常见的致病因素分述如

下：

第一节 六　　淫

六淫是风、寒、暑、湿、燥、火六种外感病邪的总称。在正常

情况下，它们本来是自然界的六种气候变化，故又名"六气"。人

类生活在自然界，对各种气候变化均有一定的适应能力，故正常

the occurrence of the six natural factors is too excessive or insufficient or unseasonable, and if the climatic variations are too rapid and violent, while the vital-*qi* of the body is weak and can not adapt to the climatic variations of nature, the six natural factors will affect the human body and cause diseases. The six natural factors under such circumstances are then called "six *yin*" (six exogenous factors). "*Yin*" here implies excess. Since six exogenous factors are unhealthy factors causing diseases, they are also called "six pathogens".

The common pathogenic characteristics of the six exogenous factors are:

① They are usually related to seasonal climate and residential environments to cause diseases. For instance, spring sees more diseases due to wind; summer, more due to summer-heat; autumn, more due to dryness; and winter, more due to cold. Living long in damp circumstances it is easy to be affected by dampness, while in high-temperature circumstances it is easy to get sunstroke.

② The six exogenous factors can either attack the body separately or simultaneously with two or more in combination to cause diseases. For example, wind-cold type of common cold and wind-cold-dampness type of arthralgia.

③ Under certain conditions the six exogenous factors can intertransform after invading the human body. For instance, pathogenic cold may transform into heat after entering the body, while in the course of time summer-heat and dampness may transform into dryness impairing *yin*,

④ The six exogenous factors cause some diseases mostly by invading the body through the skin or the mouth and nose or both, therefore diseases so caused are called "exogenous diseases".

From the viewpoint of modern medicine, besides climatic factors, diseases due to six exogenous factors also include the pathological changes caused by the effect of biological (bacteria,

的六气一般并不使人致病。如气候变化异常，六气太过或不及，或非其时而有其气，以及气候变化过于急骤，人体正气虚弱，不能适应自然界的气候变化，六气才会侵犯人体而发病。这种情况下的六气，便称为"六淫"。淫，有太过之意。由于六淫是导致疾病发生的不正之气，故又称为"六邪"。

六淫致病的共同特点是：

① 六淫致病多与季节气候、居处环境有关。如春季多风病，夏季多暑病，长夏多湿病，秋季多燥病，冬季多寒病。久居湿地多受湿，高温环境易中暑。

② 六淫邪气既可单独侵袭人体，又可两种以上同时侵犯人体而致病，如风寒感冒、风寒湿痹。

③ 六淫之邪侵入人体后，在一定条件下可以相互转化。如寒邪入里可以化热，暑湿日久可以化燥伤阴。

④ 六淫致病，多从肌表或口鼻而入，或两者同时受邪，故称"外感病"。

六淫致病，从现代医学角度看，除了气候因素外，还包括了

virus, etc.), physical, chemical and various other pathogenic factors on the human body.

In addition, there is also a doctrine called "Five Endo-pathogens" which refer to the syndromes similar to wind, cold, dampness, dryness and fire, due to the functional derangement of the viscera. For the convenience of differentiation, they are referred to as endogenous wind, endogenous cold, endogenous dampness, endogenous dryness and endogenous fire. They are discussed together with the six exogenous factors in the following.

1. Wind

Wind prevails in spring but there is wind in all the four seasons. Though diseases due to pathogenic wind occur frequently in spring they are not limited to spring only. Pathogenic wind is differentiated into exopathic wind and endogenous wind. Exopathic wind results mostly from the excess of pathogenic wind and is a very important pathogenic factor in diseases produced by exopathogens. Endogenous wind is mostly caused by the functional derangement of the liver. So the chapter "The Most Important Discussion" in *Plain Questions* (Chapter 74) says: "All tremor and dizziness due to pathogenic wind are caused by the disorder of the liver." The nature and pathogenic characteristics of pathogenic wind are as follows:

1) Pathogenic wind is apt to move and tends to rise, disperse, move upward and outward, and is thus of *yang* nature. When pathogenic wind attacks, it tends to break the barrier of skin, causing such symptoms as aversion to wind and perspiration. Pathogenic wind usually attacks the upper part of the body (head and face), skin and muscle, causing headache, dizziness, deviation of the eye and mouth and the like.

2) Pathogenic wind is apt to migrate and change. By "migrate" it means when pathogenic wind attacks the body,

生物(细菌、病毒等)、物理、化学等多种致病因素作用于人体所引起的病理变化。

此外，尚有"内生五邪"之说。是指由于脏腑功能失调所引起的类似风、寒、湿、燥、火的证候。为便于区别，将其分别称之为内风、内寒、内湿、内燥、内火。在此合并介绍。

1. 风

风为春季的主气，但四季皆有风。故风邪致病虽春季多见，但并不限于春季。风邪有外风、内风之分。外风多由于风气太过，为外感发病的一种极为重要的致病因素。内风多因肝脏功能失调所致。故《素问·至真要大论》说："诸风掉眩，皆属于肝。"风邪的性质及致病特点如下：

1) 风性善动，具有升发、向上、向外的特征，故属阳邪。

风邪为患，易使腠理开泄，出现恶风、汗出等症状。风邪侵袭，多伤及人的上部(头面)、肌表，出现头痛、头晕、口眼歪斜等。

2) 风性善行而数变。善行，是指风邪致病多病位游走不定，

the resulting symptoms or the locations of diseases tend to be unsteady and migratory. For example, in wind arthralgia the pain in the joints of the limbs is wandering. By "change" it means diseases caused by pathogenic wind usually occur rapidly and are capricious and variable. For example, a person suffering from apoplexy often faints and loses consciousness suddenly; in urticaria skin itching occurs in no fixed palces, coming here and there.

3) Domination of pathogenic wind may lead to mobility. This means the symptoms and signs of diseases due to pathogenic wind are characterized by vibration and involuntary movement, such as tremor, convulsion and vertigo.

4) Pathogenic wind is the leading pathogen causing all diseases. Wind is the most important pathogenic factor among the six exogenous factors. It is the first agent of the exogenous pathogenic factors to cause diseases. Other pathogenic factors mostly attach themselves to wind to invade the human body, as in wind-cold syndrome, wind-heat syndrome and wind-dampness syndrome.

2. Cold

Cold prevails in winter and exists also in other seasons. Pathogenic cold is differentiated into exopathic cold and endogenous cold. Exopathic cold refers to the environmental pathogenic cold; endogenous cold refers to the pathological manifestation of the deficiency of *yang-qi* and loss of warmness. The two are both differentiated and related. A body with *yang* deficiency and internal cold is liable to be affected by exopathic cold; and if exopathic cold enters the body and accumulates in the course of time without dispersion, it will impair *yang-qi* and result in endogenous cold. The nature and pathogenic characteristics of pathogenic cold are as follows:

1) Pathogenic cold is a *yin* pathgen and tends to impair *yang-qi*. Cold is of *yin* nature, so when pathogenic cold incurs

如风痹，其关节疼痛呈游走性；数变，是指风邪致病发病迅速，变幻无常，如中风患者，多卒然昏倒，不省人事；荨麻疹患者，皮肤瘙痒，发无定处，此起彼伏。

3）风性主动。是指风邪为患，其症状、体征具有动摇不定的特性，如震颤、抽搐、眩晕等。

4）风为百病之长。风是六淫中最主要的致病因素，是外邪致病的先导，其他病邪多依附于风而侵犯人体。如外感风寒、风热、风湿等。

2. 寒

寒为冬季的主气，其他季节亦可见到。寒邪有外寒、内寒之分。外寒是指寒邪外袭；内寒是机体阳气不足，失却温煦的病理反映。二者既有区别，又有联系。阳虚内寒之体，容易感受外寒，而外来寒邪侵入机体，积久不散，又能损及阳气，导致内寒。寒邪的性质及致病特点如下：

1）寒为阴邪，易伤阳气。寒性属阴，故寒邪致病，最易损

diseases it is most liable to impair the *yang-qi* of the human body. For example, when pathogenic cold invades the superficial portion of the body and the defensive *yang* is checked, aversion to cold may appear; when pathogenic cold attacks directly the spleen and stomach and the middle-*jiao yang* is thus impaired, abdominal cold-pain may come on.

2) Pathogenic cold is coagulative and obstructive in nature. When pathogenic cold attacks the human body, it may block or coagulate *qi* and blood in the channels and impede their flow, causing various kinds f pain.

3) Cold causes constriction. When pathogenic cold enters the body it may cause the functional activities of *qi* to constrict and cause the muscular striae, channels and collaterals and tendons to contract and thus incur contracture and spasm. For instance, when pathogenic cold attacks the body surface, the sweat pores and muscular striae will be closed and contracted, the defensive *yang* will be stagnated and prevented from going outward, bringing on aversion to cold with fever and anhidrosis; if pathogenic cold invades the channels and collaterals and joints, there will occur muscular cramp and retarded flexion and extension of joints.

3. Summer-heat

Summer-heat prevails in summer. It is transformed from fire and heat. Summer heat is a pure exopathogen, Its nature and pathogenic characteristics are as follows:

1) Summer-heat is a *yang* pathogen and is scorching hot in nature. Summer-heat is transformed from summer's scorching heat which is of *yang* nature, and is thus a *yang* pathogen. When pathogenic summer-heat attacks the body, there tends to appear such symptoms as high fever, upset, flushed face and full rapid pulse.

2) Summer-heat tends to rise and disperse. It exhausts *qi* and impairs the body fluid. Pathogenic summer-heat usually

伤人体阳气。如寒邪袭表，卫阳被遏，可见恶寒；寒邪直中脾胃，中阳受损，可见脘腹冷痛。

2）寒性凝滞。凝滞，即凝结、阻滞不通之意。寒邪伤人，可使经脉气血凝滞，运行不畅而出现各种疼痛。

3）寒性收引。收引，即收缩牵引的意思。寒邪侵入人体，易使气机收敛，腠理、经络、筋脉收缩而挛急。如寒客肌表，毛窍、肌腠收缩，卫阳郁闭，出现恶寒、发热而无汗；寒客经络、关节，则拘挛作痛，屈伸不利。

3. 暑

暑为夏季的主气，乃火热所化。暑纯属外邪。其性质及致病特点如下：

1）暑为阳邪，其性炎热。暑为夏季火热之气所化，火热属阳，故暑为阳邪。暑邪伤人，多出现壮热、心烦、面赤、脉洪等阳热症状。

2）暑性升散，耗气伤津。暑邪致病，易使腠理开泄而多汗。

brings on diseases by opening the striae of skin and the body fluid, resulting in thirst and desire for drinking, dryness of the lips and tongue, and scanty dark urine. Together with profuse perspiration, *qi* is also lost with the body fluid, resulting in deficiency of *qi* and causing shortness of breath, lassitude, and even sudden fainting and loss of consciousness.

3) Summer-heat is usually accompanied with dampness. Summer is a hot, rainy season, so pathogenic summer-heat is usually accompanied with dampness to cause diseases. Apart from such summer-heat symptoms as fever, thirst and the like, the clinical manifestations are often accompanied with lassitude of the limbs, chest distress, vomiting, nausea and sticky loose stool.

4. Dampness

Dampness prevails in late summer. Late summer is a time when summer is changing into autumn, a season when dampness is the most exuberant in the year, so in this season it is easy to contract diseases due to dampness, which may also incur diseases in other seasons. Pathagenic dampness is differentiated into exopathic dampness and endogenous dampness. Exopathic dampness is usually due to damp climate, wading in water or being caught in a rain, as well as damp dwelling environments, Endogenous dampness is usually caused by the dysfunction of the spleen in transportation leading to the impairment of water metabolism. Exopathic and endogenous dampness can influence each other and are interdependent. The nature and pathogenic characteristics of pathogenic dampness are as follows:

1) Dampness is heavy and turbid in nature. Heaviness in a damp disease is usually marked by heavy sensations as lassitude, heavy sensation of the head and body, and aching and sluggishness of the limbs. As turbidness is concerned, a damp disease is usually marked by turbid excreta and secreta such as

汗出过多则伤津，出现口渴喜饮、唇干舌燥、尿赤短少等。在大量汗出的同时，往往气随津泄而致气虚，出现气短乏力，甚则突然昏倒，不省人事。

3）暑多挟湿。暑季酷热多雨，故暑邪为病，多挟湿邪。临床表现除发热、烦渴等暑热症状外，常兼见四肢困倦、胸闷呕恶、大便溏泄不爽等。

4．湿

湿为长夏的主气，时当夏秋之交，为一年中湿气最盛的季节，故易患湿病，但其他季节也可发病。湿邪为病，有外湿、内湿之分。外湿多因气候潮湿、涉水淋雨、居处潮湿所致；内湿则是由于脾失健运、水湿内停而生。外湿、内湿常互相影响，互为因果。湿邪的性质及致病特点如下：

1）湿性重浊。重，即沉重或重着之意。指湿邪为病，常有头身困重、四肢酸懒等沉重感觉。浊，即秽浊之意。指湿邪为患，多表现为排泄物和分泌物秽浊不洁，如面垢眵多、大便溏泄或有

much facial filth and eye secretions, loose stool or mucous stool with pus and blood, turbid urine, excessive leukorrhea and turbid pyogenic fluid.

2) Dampness is viscous and lingering in nature, which is manifested in two aspects: in one aspect, the symptoms of a damp disease are usually of slimy and greasy feature, for instance, slimy and greasy fur, mucous difficult stool and difficult urination; in the other aspect, a damp disease has a long course and is often lingering and difficult to cure, as can be seen in damp arthralgia, eczema and damp-warm syndrome.

3) Dampness tends to go downward. The symptoms of a damp disease are mostly found in the lower part of the body, such as leukorrhagia, stranguria with turbid urine, diarrhea and dysentery.

4) Dampness is a *yin* pathogen which tends to obstruct the functional activities of *qi* and impair *yang-qi*. Dampness is heavy and turbid, and is similar to water in nature, thus is defined as a *yin* pathogen. When pathogenic dampness attacks, it is most liable to lead to the disorder of the ascending or descending ability and digestive functions of *qi*. For example, when there is retention of dampness in the epigastrium and impediment in the functional activities of *qi*, there will appear distress in the chest; when dampness blocks the spleen and stomach and cause dysfunction of the spleen in water circulation as well as the disturbance of the spleen-*qi* to ascend and the stomach-*qi* to descend, there will appear anorexia, epigastric distress, nausea, vomiting and loose stool. As dampness is a *yin* pathogen which tends to impair *yang-qi*, when it disturbs the spleen, the spleen-*yang* will be insufficient, then there will be dysfunction of the spleen in fluid transportation and transformation and retention of dampness within the body, resulting in diarrhea, edema, difficult urination and the like.

脓血粘液、小便混浊、白带过多及脓水秽浊等。

2）湿性粘滞。粘，即粘腻；滞，即停滞。湿性粘滞主要表现在两方面：一是湿病症状多粘腻不爽，如舌苔粘腻、大便粘滞不爽、小便涩滞不畅等；二是湿邪为病，病程较长，缠绵难愈，如湿痹、湿疹、湿温病等。

3）湿性趋下。湿邪为病，其症状多见于下部，如带下、淋浊、泄痢等。

4）湿为阴邪，易阻气机，损伤阳气。湿性重浊，其性类水，故属阴邪。湿邪为患，最易阻滞气机，使其升降失常。如湿阻胸膈，气机不畅，则胸闷；湿困脾胃，运化失职，升降失常，则纳呆、脘闷、呕恶、便溏。由于湿为阴邪，易伤人阳气，湿邪困脾，脾阳不振，运化无权，水湿停聚，从而出现泄泻、水肿、小便不利等。

5. Dryness

Dryness prevails in autumn. Autumn is a dry season with shortage of water. Dryness diseases are most likely to occur in such a season. Pathogenic dryness can be divided into exopathic dryness and endogenous dryness. Diseases caused by exopathic dryness are mostly due to affection by environmental dry pathogens. Exopathic dryness is subdivided into warm-dryness and cool-dryness. Warm-dryness is mostly found in early autumn, formed by the remaining heat of late summer and pathogenic dryness in combination. Cool-dryness is mostly found in late autumn, formed by the pathogenic cold of approaching winter and pathogenic dryness in combination. When exopathic dryness attacks the human body it usually invades from the mouth and nose and afflicts the defensive qi and the lung, forming exterior syndrome. Endogenous dryness mostly results from the exhaustion of essence and blood by lingering diseases, the consumption of body fluid by febrile diseases, improper treatment and loss of blood. The nature and pathogenic characteristics of pathogenic dryness are as follows:

1) Pathogenic dryness is dry and tends to impair the body fluid. When pathogenic dryness attacks, various forms of symptoms and signs presenting deficiency of body fluid and dryness are most likely to appear, such as dryness in the mouth and nose, dryness of the throat, thirst, dryness of the skin and even rhagas, oliguria and constipation.

2) Pathogenic dryness tends to impair the lung. The lung is a delicate organ which prefers moisture to dryness and is vulnerable to the attack of dryness. The lung is related to the skin and hair of the body surface and has its specific orifice in the nose, so pathogenic dryness usually attacks through the mouth and nose and is most liable to impair the lung, causing such symptoms as dryness of the nose and throat, dry cough with little phlegm, dyspnea or asthma and chest pain.

5. 燥

燥为秋季的主气。此时气候干燥，水分亏乏，故多燥病。燥邪有外燥、内燥之分。外燥多因感受外界燥邪而发病，其中又有温燥、凉燥之别。温燥多见于初秋，由夏之余热与燥邪相合而成；凉燥多由近冬寒邪与燥邪相合而生。外燥伤人，多自口鼻而入，侵犯肺卫，形成表证。内燥多因病久精血内夺、热病耗伤津液以及误治、失血所致。燥邪的性质及致病特点如下：

1) 燥邪干涩，易伤津液。燥邪为病，最易出现各种津亏干涩症状和体征，如口鼻干燥、咽干口渴、皮肤干涩甚则皲裂、小便短少、大便干结等。

2) 燥易伤肺。肺为娇脏，喜润而恶燥。肺外合皮毛，开窍于鼻，故燥邪伤人，多从口鼻而入，最易伤肺，出现鼻干咽燥、干咳少痰及喘息胸痛等症。

6. Fire

Fire is different from warm and heat though they are of the same nature. Warm and heat are both referred to as pathogens, they are different only in degree and are the same in nature. So they are often mentioned together. Fire has two meanings: one refers to the vital-*qi* in the human body and is called "junior fire" in *The Yellow Emperor's Canon of Internal Medicine*; the other refers to a pathogen called "sthenic fire" in *The Yellow Emperor's Canon of Internal Medicine*.

Pathogenic fire is divided into exopathic fire and endogenous fire. Affection by exopathic fire is mostly caused direct by the invasion of external pathogenic warm and heat; endogenous fire usually results from the excess of visceral *yang-qi*, as Zhu Danxi said: "The excess of *qi* is fire." In addition, affections by various exopathogens such as wind, cold, dampness and dryness or mental irritation can all transform into fire under certain conditions. The nature and pathogenic characteristics of pathogenic fire are as follows:

1) Fire tends to burn and scorch. When pathogenic fire causes diseases, there often appear such symptoms as high fever, flushed face, blood-shot eyes, aversion to heat, desire for the cool, constipation, dark scanty urine and red tongue with yellow fur.

2) Fire tends to flare up. Symptoms caused by pathogenic fire tend to appear on the upper part of the body, for instance, on the head and face. For example, when heart-fire flares up, reddened tongue-tip tends to appear; when stomach-fire exuberates and flares up, painful swollen gum may appear; when liver-fire flares up, congested swollen eyes with pain may occur.

3) Fire tends to impair the body fluid and consume *qi*. When pathogenic fire attacks, it tends to force the body fluid to leak out and scorch the fluid, impairing and consuming *yin* fluid, so it is often accompanied with symptoms of fluid impair-

6. 火

火与温热，虽性质相同，但有区别。温与热均指病邪而言，二者仅程度不同。并无本质差异，故中医常温热并称。火有两种含义：一是指人体的正气，《黄帝内经》称之为"少火"；二是指病邪，《黄帝内经》称之为"壮火"。

火邪亦有内外之分。属外感者，多是直接感受温热邪气之侵袭；属内生者，常因脏腑阳气过盛而成，即朱丹溪所说："气有余便是火"。此外，感受风、寒、湿、燥等各种外邪，或精神刺激，在一定条件下皆可化火。火邪的性质及致病特点如下：

1) 火性燔灼。燔，即燃烧，灼，即烧烫。火邪致病，多见高热、面红目赤、恶热喜凉、便秘尿赤、舌红苔黄等证候。

2) 火性炎上。火邪致病，证候多表现在人体的上部，如头面部位。若心火上炎，则见舌尖红；胃火炽盛，可见齿龈肿痛；肝火上炎，常见目赤肿痛。

3) 火易伤津耗气。火邪为患，最易迫津外泄，消灼津液，耗伤阴津，故常兼有口渴喜饮、咽干口燥、小便短赤、大便干结

ment such as thirst with desire for drinking, dryness of the throat and mouth, dark scanty urine and constipation. Pathogenic fire is most liable to impair the vital-*qi* of the body, so diseases caused by fire are often accompanied with such symptoms as deficiency of *qi*, disinclination to talk and lassitude.

4) Fire tends to promote the production of liver wind and accelerate the circulation of blood. When pathogenic fire enters the body, it scorches the liver-*yin*, depriving the tendon and muscle of their nourishment and leading to the up-stirring of liver wind, causing high fever, convulsion, anoopsia, stiffness of the neck and opisthotonus. Pathogenic fire may accelerate the flow of blood which may scorch the channels and collaterals and even force the blood to go astray, causing various bleeding symptoms such as hemoptysis, nosebleed, hemafecia, hematuria, macule and papule, and metrorrhagia and metrostaxis.

5) Fire tends to cause carbuncles and sores. When pathogenic fire enters the blood system, it may accumulate in a local part, rotting the flesh and spoiling the blood to form carbuncles, sores and other infections, manifested as local redness, swelling, heat and pain, even suppuration and ulceration.

6) Fire tends to irritate the heart and spirit. The heart's main function is to govern vessels and store spirit. When pathogenic fire attacks, it is most liable to irritate the heart and spirit. In mild cases there may appear upset and insomnia; in severe cases mania, restlessness, unconsciousness and delirium may occur.

Section 2

Epidemic Pathogenic Factor

Epidemic pathogenic factor is a kind of pathogen of strong infectivity. In traditional Chinese medical literature, it is also

等津伤症状。火邪最能损伤人体的正气，故火邪致病，还可兼见少气懒言、肢体乏倦等气虚症状。

4）火易生风动血。火邪侵入人体，往往灼伤肝阴，使筋脉失去濡养，而致肝风内动，出现高热、抽搐、目睛上视、颈项强直、角弓反张等。火邪为患，可加速血行，易灼伤脉络，甚则迫血妄行，出现咯血、衄血、便血、尿血、斑疹、崩漏等各种出血病症。

5）火易致痈疡。火邪侵入血分，可聚于局部，腐肉败血，发为痈肿疮疡，表现为局部红肿热痛，甚至化脓溃烂。

6）火易扰心神。心主血脉而藏神，火邪为患，最易扰乱心神。轻者心烦、失眠；重者狂躁妄动、神昏谵语等。

第二节　疠　气

疠气是一类传染性极强的病邪。在中医文献中，又有"瘟疫"、

referred to as "pestilence", "epidemic toxin", "morbid air", "unusual evil", "absurd evil" and so forth.

Epidemic pathogenic factor is a kind of minute pathogenic substance (pathogenic microorganism) that can not be observed directly by the human sensory organs. It usually invades the human body through the mouth and nose. The discovery of epidemic pathogenic factor is a magnificant stride in the etiology of traditional Chinese medicine. Sudden onset, severe conditions of illness, similar manifestations, strong infectivity and strong epidemicity are characteristics of epidemic pathogenic factor, which can be seen in fulminant dysentery, diphtheria, scarlet fever, smallpox, cholera, plague and so on. These have actually covered many of infectious diseases in modern medicine.

The attack of epidemic pathogenic factor is usually related to unusual climate such as long droughts, floods, extreme heat as well as air pollution, water or food contamination and failure of timely effective prevention and isolation.

People are often immunized after contracting epidemic diseases; in some cases life-long immunity may be acquired. According to this fact, traditional Chinese medicine developed the method of "human variolation" as early as around the 10th century A.D., thus became the founder of artificial immunity in the world. At present, Chinese health organizations at various levels are widely practising artificial immunity to prevent diseases and have effected remarkable reduction of the morbidity of infectious diseases among which such fulminating infectious diseases as smallpox, cholera and plague were eradicated long before.

Clinical practice shows that traditional Chinese medicine and medicinal herbs have a satisfactory therapeutic effect on may infectious diseases such as influenza, bacillary dysentery and infectious hepatitis, and have been highly evaluated.

"疫毒"、"戾气"、"异气"、"乖戾之气"等名称。

疠气是一类人的感官所不能直接观察到的微小致病物质（病原微生物），且多由口鼻侵入人体。疠气的发现，是中医病因学的重大突破。疠气致病，具有发病急骤、病情较重、症状相似、传染性强、易于流行等特点，如疫痢、白喉、烂喉丹痧、天花、霍乱、鼠疫等。这些实际上包括了现代医学中的许多传染病。

疠气为患，多与气候反常，如天旱、涝灾、酷热等，空气、水源或食物受到污染，以及没有及时做好预防隔离工作有关。

患疫疠病后常有免疫性，有的获得终身免疫，不再复患。中医根据这一特点，早在公元十世纪前后就创造了"人痘接种术"，成为世界人工免疫的先驱。目前，中国各级卫生机构广泛开展人工免疫预防疾病，使传染病发病率显著下降。其中，天花、霍乱、鼠疫等烈性传染病早已绝迹。

临床实践证明，中医药对流感、菌痢、传染性肝炎等多种传染病疗效甚佳，受到了广泛的重视。

Section 3

Parasites

A long time ago traditional Chinese medicine realized that parasites can cause diseases. For example, the Eastern Han Dynasty physician Zhang Zhongjing discussed "colic caused by ascaris" (biliary ascariasis) in his *Treatise on Febrile Diseases* (3rd century A.D.); in the Sui Dynasty, Chao Yuanfang's *General Treatise on the Etiology and Symptomatology of Diseases* (610 A.D.) had already had relatively detailed records of oxyuriasis and taeniasis, holding that the predisposing factor is unhygienic diet, and that taeniasis caused by eating undercooked beef. Traditional Chinese medicine calls schistosomiasis "noxious water disease", believing it to be caused by drinking contaminated pool water.

The clinical manifestations of various parasite are different. Ascarides parasitize in the intestinal tract, thus abdominal pains frequently occur: if ascarides run up into the biliary tract, they may cause colic. Patients with ancylostomiasis usually look sallow and emaciated and have paroxia. Patients suffering from oxyuriasis often complain about anus and perinea pruritus, and white minute linear oxyurids can be found instantly in these parts. The symptoms of taeniasis are relatively slight. Patients go to seek medical advice usually because white bandshaped imaginal proglottides are found in their feces. Hepatosplenomegaly and impeded circulation of blood caused by schistosomiasis lead to the accumulation and retention of fluid in the abdomen, forming "tympanites". Chinese medicinal herbs are safe and reliable in treating parasitoses.

第三节 寄 生 虫

中医早已认识到寄生虫能引起疾病，如东汉医家 张 仲 景 在

《伤寒论》中就论述了"蛔厥"（胆道蛔虫）的证治。至隋代，在巢元

方的《诸病源候论》中，对蛲虫病、绦虫病已有较详细的记载，认

为其发病原因是饮食不洁，而绦虫病是因食用不熟牛肉所致。中

医将血吸虫病称为"水毒"，认为是因饮用被污染的池水而致。

各种寄生虫病的临床特征不同。蛔虫寄生于肠道，腹痛时作；

蛔虫上窜胆道，可致蛔厥。钩虫病常表现为面黄肌瘦、嗜食异物。

蛲虫病患者常主诉肛门、会阴瘙痒，并可在这些部位直接找到白

色细小线状蛲虫。绦虫病症状较轻，常因粪便中发现白色带状成

虫节片而就医。血吸虫病因其肝脾肿大、血行不畅而致水液停聚

于腹，形成"蛊胀"。中医药治疗寄生虫病安全而可靠。

Section 4

Internal Injury by Seven Emotions

Seven emotions refer to the seven kinds of emotional reactions, namely: joy, anger, melancholy, anxiety, grief, fear and terror, being the different responses of the human body to the environmental stimuli. In general circumstances, these are within the normal range of mental activities and will not cause diseases, but when sudden, violent or long-term persistent emotional stimuli occur beyond the adaptability and endurance of the body, they will cause the functional disorder and derangement of *zang-fu* organs (or viscera and bowels) and *qi*, [and the emotional stimuli will then become pathogenic factors, which is referred to as internal injury by seven emotions.

1. Relationship between Seven Emotions and the Viscera

Traditional Chinese medicine holds that human mental activities are closely related with the viscera. "The Principle of *Yin-Yang* Doctrine and Its Relation with Natural Things or Phenomena", Chapter 5 in *Plain Questions* says: "Man has five viscera which may bring on five moods (visceral-*qi*) to produce joy, anger, grief, melancholy and fear". It also believes that certain viscus is related to certain emotional activity, i.e. the heart is related to joy, liver to anger, spleen to anxiety, the lung to melancholy and the kidney to fear. Only by acting on the corresponding viscus can the environmental emotional stimuli evoke specific emotional response.

第四节　七　情　内　伤

七情，即喜、怒、忧、思、悲、恐、惊七种情志变化，是人体对客观事物的不同反映。在一般情况下，属正常精神活动范围，不会使人致病。但突然、强烈或长期、持久的情志刺激，超过了人体的适应能力和耐受程度，就会使人脏腑功能紊乱，气机失调而发病。这时，情志刺激就成为致病因素，称为七情内伤。

1. 七情与内脏的关系

中医认为，人的精神活动与内脏密切相关，如《素问·阴阳应象大论》说："人有五脏化五气，以生喜怒悲忧恐"。并且还认为，某一内脏常与某一情志活动有关，即心在志为喜，肝在志为怒，脾在志为思，肺在志为忧，肾在志为恐。外界的情志刺激，只有作用于相应的内脏，才能表现为特定的情志反映。

2. Pathogenic Characteristics of Seven Emotions

The seven emotions are different from the six exogenous factors in causing diseases. The six exogenous factors usually invade the body through the skin, mouth and nose, and it is exterior syndrome that mostly appears at the early stage of the onset. However, the seven emotions directly affect the corresponding viscus to bring on diseases, as the chapter "The Principle of *Yin-Yang* Doctrine and its Relation with Natural Things or Phenomena" (Chapter 5) in *Plain Questions* says: "Anger impairs the liver", "Joy impairs the heart", "Anxiety impairs the spleen", "Melancho'y impairs the lung", "Fear impairs the kidney". As the heart controls mental activities and is the arch-governor of the five *zang*- organs (or the five viscera) and six *fu*- organs (or the six bowels), the chapter "Questions about Pathogens of Yawn and Others" (Chapter 28) in *Miraculous Pivot* says: "Excessive grief, sorrow, worry and melancholy will affect the heart, when the heart is affected, the five *zang*-organs and six *fu*-organs will all be stirred in accordance."

The seven emotions mainly affect the functional activities of the visceral-*qi* to impair the viscera, as the chapter "Discussion on Etiology and Pathogenesis of Pain" (Chapter 39) in *Plain Questions* says: "Rage causes adverse upward flow of the liver-*qi*, excessive joy relaxes the heart-*qi*, excessive sorrow leads to the consumption of *qi*, fear causes the sinking of the kidney-*qi*,... fright interrupts the flow of *qi*, anxiety causes the stagnation of the spleen-*qi*,"

Emotional stimuli may cause the functional derangement of visceral-*qi* which can lead to changes of emotional moods, as the chapter "Discussion on the Important Basis of Vitality" (Chapter 8) in *Miraculous Pivot* says: "The deficiency of the liver-*qi* causes fear, whereas the excess of the liver-*qi* will cause anger." "The deficiency of the heart-*qi* causes grief, whereas

2．七情致病的特点

七情致病与六淫不同。六淫侵袭人体，多由皮肤及口鼻而入，发病之初多见表证。而七情致病，则是直接影响相应的内脏而发病。如《素问·阴阳应象大论》说："怒伤肝"、"喜伤心"、"思伤脾"、"忧伤肺"、"恐伤肾"。由于心主神志，为五脏六腑之大主，故《灵枢·口问》说："悲哀愁忧则心动，心动则五脏六腑皆摇。"

七情伤及内脏，主要是影响脏腑的气机。如《素问·举痛论》说："怒则气上，喜则气缓，悲则气消，恐则气下，……惊则气乱，……思则气结。"

情志刺激可以引起脏腑气机失调，而脏腑气机失调又可出现不同的情志改变，如《灵枢·本神》说："肝气虚则恐，实则怒"，"心

the excess of the heart-*qi* will cause ceaseless laughing".

The seven emotions can not only cause diseases but also aggravate them.   In the course of many diseases, the condition of illness often deteriorates as the result of severe fluctuation of the patients' moods of emotions.   So traditional Chinese medicine pays great attention to the mental consolation and care the patients to prompt the diseases to turn toward a favourable side.

Section 5

Diet, Work and Rest

Diet, work and rest are the fundamental conditions for human beings to live and maintain good health.   Improper diet and maladjustment of work and rest will affect the physiological functions of the viscera and reduce the organism's resistance to diseases, thus becoming pathogenic factors.

1. Improper Diet

It includes abnormal ingestion, unhygienic diet and food preference.

1) Abnormal Ingestion   It is wise to eat an appropriate amount of food.   Excessive hunger and overfeeding can both give rise to diseases.   Excessive hunger, i.e. inadequate ingestion, results in an inadequate intake for the transformation into *qi* and blood and eventually leads to the deficiency of *qi* and blood to bring on diseases.   For instance, the chapter "Five Flavours" (Chapter 56) in *Miraculous Pivot* says: "No food ingestion for half a day will result in the decline of *qi*, and for one day in the deficiency of *qi*."   Meanwhile, the decline and deficiency of *qi* and blood will cripple the resistance to the attack of exopathogens.   Overfeeding beyond the normal digestive

气虚则悲，实则笑不休"。

七情既可致病，又可加重病情。在许多疾病的过程中，病情常因较剧烈的情绪波动而恶化。故中医十分重视对病人的精神安慰与调护，以促使疾病向好的方向转化。

第五节　饮食、劳逸

饮食、劳动和休息，是人类赖以生存和维持健康的基本条件，但如果饮食不节，或劳逸失度，就会影响脏腑的生理功能，降低机体的抗病能力，成为致病因素。

1．饮食不节

饮食不节包括饥饱失常、饮食不洁和饮食偏嗜三方面。

1）饥饱失常　饮食以适量为宜，过饥、过饱均可致病。过饥，即摄食不足，则气血生化之源不足，终致气血衰少而为病。如《灵枢·五味》说："谷不入，半日则气衰，一日则气少矣。"同时，气血衰少则抗病能力减弱，易受外邪侵袭。过饱，即饮食过量，

ability, i.e. hyperphagia, can also give rise to diseases by indigestion and retendtion of food in the middle-*jiao*, manifested as abdominal distension and fullness, eructation with fetid odor and acid regurgitation, anorexia, vomiting, diarrhea with stinking and filthy stool, etc., as the chapter "Discussion on Arthralgia-Syndrome" (Chapter 43) in *Plain Questions* says: "Excessive diet impairs the intestines and stomach." As children have weak function of the spleen and stomach and have no sense of proper diet, they are more liable to fall ill.

2) Unhygienic Diet　Unhygienic diet can cause many kinds of gastro-intestinal diseases, manifested as diarrhea, abdominal pain, vomiting, purulent and bloody stool and the like, as well as various kinds of parasitos s. Rotten or poisonous food may result in food poisoning. In slight cases there may appear vomiting, diarrhea and abdominal pain; in severe cases, there will be the impairment of body fluid and loss of *yang*, leading to depression of the socket of the eyeball and cold limbs.

3) Food Preference　Man is nourished by food. Only through an appropriate mixture of food can man acquire various necessary nutrients. Any food preference may cause the derangement of *yin* and *yang*, nutritional deficiency and give rise to diseases. For example, preference for cold and uncooked food is liable to impair the middle-*jiao yang*; preference for dry hot food is liable to produce stomach-heat; a rich fatty diet is liable to cause carbuncles and furuncles. Addiction to one of the five flavours (sour, bitter, sweet, acid and salty) can also give rise to diseases, as the chapter "The Close Relationship bewteen Human Activity and Nature" (Chapter 3) in *Plain Questions* says "Excessive sour nourished the liver-*qi* and leads to the exhaustion of the spleen-*qi*; excessive salty flavour leads to large consumption of *qi* of bones, myoatrophy and depression of the heart-*qi*; excessive sweetness causes sickness of the heart-*qi*, dyspnea and chest fullness, dark complexion and an unbalance of the kidney-*qi*; excessive bitterness

超过了正常的消化能力，也会因食积中焦而发病，表现为脘腹胀满、嗳腐吞酸、厌食呕吐、泻下臭秽等，故《素问·痹论》说："饮食自倍，肠胃乃伤。"小儿由于脾胃尚弱，不知饥饱，更易患病。

2）饮食不洁　饮食不洁可引起多种胃肠道疾病（表现为呕吐、泄泻、腹痛、便脓血等）或各种寄生虫病。若误食腐败变质或有毒食物，可引起食物中毒，轻者吐泻腹痛，重者伤津亡阳，出现眼窝下陷、四肢厥冷等。

3）饮食偏嗜　人以五谷为养，饮食应适当调配，才能获得各种必需的营养。任何偏嗜，都可造成阴阳失调或营养缺乏而致病。如偏食生冷，易伤中阳；偏食燥热，易生胃热；膏粱厚味，易发痈疔。偏嗜五味，亦可致病。如《素问·生气通天论》说："味过于酸，肝气以津，脾气乃绝；味过于咸，大骨气劳，短肌，心气抑；味过于甘，心气喘满，色黑，肾气不衡；味过于苦，脾气

leads to failure of the spleen-qi to transport and transform nutrients and depression of the stomach-qi: excessive pungent flavour leads to flaccidity of tendon and muscle and loss of spirit." In addition, beriberi, night blindness and goiter are all results of addiction to one of the five flavours and malnutrition.

2. Maladjustment of Work and Rest

Maladjustment of work and rest includes overstrain and overrest.

1) Overstrain   Overstrain includes physical overstrain, mental overstrain and sexual overstrain.

(1)Physical overstrain: Referring to the overstrain from physical labour.   The chapter "Discussion on Etiology, Pathogenesis and Characteristics of Various Pains" (Chapter 39) in *Plain Questions* says: "Over-exertion results in qi exhaustion." In mild cases there may appear lassitude, deficiency of qi and disinclination to talk and mental fatigue; in severe cases, there will be injury of tendon, muscle and bone, causing lumbago, arthralgia and myalgia of the limbs.

(2)Mental overstrain: Referring to the overstrain from mental labour.   Mental overstrain may consume and impair the heart-blood and impair the spleen-qi, causing palpitation, amnesia, insomnia, dreaminess, anorexia, abdominal distension, loose stool and so on.

(3)Sexual overstrain: Referring to the intemperance in sexual life.   Proper sexual life does no harm to health and instead is helpful to sleep and rest; but indulgence in sexual activities can exhaust and impair the kidney essence, causing lassitude in the loins and knees, dizziness, tinnitus and listlessness; and impotence, spermatorrhea or no ejaculation in males, menoxenia and leukorrhagia in females.

2) Overrest   Overrest refers to excessive rest and comfort. No labour and exercises can lead to impeded circulation of qi and blood, flaccidity and crispness of tendon. muscle and bone,

不濡，胃气乃厚，味过于辛，筋脉沮弛，精神乃央。"此外，脚气病、夜盲病、瘿瘤病等，亦是偏嗜五味、营养不全的结果。

2．劳逸失度

劳逸失度包括过劳和过逸两个方面。

1）过劳　包括劳力过度、劳神过度和房劳过度。

（1）劳力过度：是指体力劳动过度。《素问·举痛论》说："劳则气耗。"轻者疲倦无力、少气懒言、精神疲惫；重者筋骨肌肉损伤，出现腰痛、肢体关节肌肉疼痛等。

（2）劳神过度：是指脑力劳动过度。如劳神过度，耗伤心血，损伤脾气，可出现心悸、健忘、失眠、多梦、纳呆、腹胀和便溏等。

（3）房劳过度：是指性生活过频。有节制的性生活，不但不损伤身体，反而有助于睡眠和休息。但如房事不节，可耗伤肾精，出现腰膝酸软、眩晕耳鸣、精神萎靡，男子阳痿、滑泄或不射精，女子月经不调、带下等。

2）过逸　是指过度安逸。不劳动、不锻炼，可使气血不畅，

and the stagnation of the spleen and stomach, manifested as listlessness, loss of appetite, lassitude, shortness of breath on exertion, palpitation or obesity. It also cripples the body's resistance to diseases and makes the body susceptible to the attack or exopathogens.

Section 6

Surgical Trauma

Surgical trauma includes gunshot wound, incised wound, traumatic injuries (including injuries by knife and spear, fall and stumble, contusion, stabbing and abrasion and sport injuries), injuries by heavy load, twist, sprain and wrench, burns and scalds, and bites by insects and beasts. In slight cases there may be wound, bleeding, swelling and pain of the skin, muscle and other tissues, or bone fractures and joint dislocation. In severe cases there may be injury of internal organs and blood vessels, causing visceral bleeding, blood stasis, dysfunction, hemorrhage, *yin* and *yang* depletion, and even death.

Section 7

Retention of Phlegm and Fluid, and Blood Stasis

Retention of phlegm and fluid and blood stasis are both pathological products in the body which form in the course of illness. When they are formed, they can in turn act, directly or indirectly, on certain tissue or organ of the human body, causing new pathological changes, forming various different syndromes. So they are also one group of pathogenic factors.

筋骨柔脆，脾胃呆滞，表现为精神不振，食少乏力，动则气短、

心悸，或发为臃肿，并使抗病能力降低，易受外邪侵袭。

第六节　外　伤

外伤包括枪伤、金刃伤、跌打损伤、持重努伤、烧烫伤及虫

兽伤等。轻者可引起皮肤、肌肉等组织破创、出血、肿痛，或骨

折、脱臼等；重者可损伤内脏、血脉，造成内脏出血、瘀血、功

能障碍、亡血、亡阴、亡阳，甚至死亡。

第七节　痰饮、瘀血

痰饮和瘀血都是人体在疾病过程中所形成的病理产物。其形

成后，又能直接或间接地作用于人体的某一组织、器官，引起新

的病理改变，形成各种不同的证候，故亦属致病因素之一。

1. Retention of Phlegm and Fluid

Retention of phlegm and fluid is characterized by accumulation of dampness as a pathological product resulting from disturbances of water metabolism. Traditional Chinese medicine classifies the thicker turbid dampness as phlegm and the thinner clearer one as fluid. Retention of phlegm and fluid is further differentiated into concrete and formless ones. Concrete retention of phlegm and fluid refers to the visible, palpable and audible parenchymatous phlegm and fluid, whereas formless retention of phlegm and fluid refers to the various conditions caused by the retention, such as dizziness, chest tightness, manic-depressive psynchosis, subcutaneous nodule and scrofula, characterized by greasy fur and slippery pulse. It is so called "formless phlegm" because this kind of "phlegm" only shows its symptoms but has no concrete form and can be cured by methods of eliminating phlegm.

Retention of phlegm and fluid is mostly due to affection by the six exogenous factors or improper diet, or internal damage by the seven emotions. These etiological factors bring forth dysfunction of *qi* of the lung, spleen, kidney and the *sanjiao* with disturbance of water-fluid metabolism, resulting in accumulation of fluid within the body. Once the retention is formed, it can follow *qi* to circulate, inward into the viscera and outward to the skin, muscle, tendon and bone. It can actually reach everywhere and cause a number of diseases. For instance, stagnation of phlegm in the lung may cause cough with dyspnea and expectoration; phlegm stagnation in the heart may cause palpitation and chest oppression; mental confusion due to the invasion of phlegm to the heart may cause coma and dementia; accumulation of phlegm in the middle-*jiao* may cause epigastric fullness, vomiting, nausea and dizziness; stagnation of phlegm in the channels and collaterals may lead to numbness of the limbs, difficult flexion and exten-

1. 痰饮

痰饮是水液代谢障碍所形成的病理产物。中医将其较稠浊的称为痰，清稀的称为饮。痰饮又有有形、无形之分。有形之痰乃指视之可见，触之可及，闻之有声的实质性痰浊和饮液；无形之痰则是指因痰饮所引起的各种病证，如眩晕、胸闷、癫狂、痰核、瘰疬等，并以苔腻、脉滑为特征。由于这种"痰"只见其症，不见其形，而用治痰法又可使其痊愈，故称之为"无形之痰"。

痰饮多因外感六淫，或饮食、七情内伤，使肺、脾、肾及三焦气化功能失职，水液代谢发生障碍，停聚体内而成。痰饮形成后，可随气流行，内而脏腑，外至皮肉、筋骨，无处不到，从而形成多种病证。如痰滞在肺，可见咳喘、咯痰；痰阻于心，可有心悸、胸闷；痰迷心窍，可致神昏、痴呆；痰浊中阻,可觉脘闷、呕恶、眩晕；痰留经络，可致肢体麻木、屈伸不利，甚至半身不遂；痰在肌肉、筋骨，可致阴疽、流注；痰结聚皮下，可形成痰

sion, and even hemiplegia; stagnation of phlegm in the tendon,

Pathogenic fluid has different manifestation in accordance with its stagnation in different parts of the body. As *Synopsis of the Golden Chamber* says: "A person who used to be in good health is now very thin; if fluid flows in the intestines and makes audible noises, we call it phlegm retention (in the narrower sense); if fluid flows in the hypochondrium and causes hypochondriac pain with cough and spitting, we call it pleural effusion; if fluid circulates in the four limbs, causing anhidrosis when perspiration is expected and leading to pain of the body, we call it diffuse fluid-retention; when there is cough with dyspnea, shortness of breath, inability to sleep and edema, we call it excessive fluid in the chest and hypochondrium."

2. Blood Stasis

Blood stasis is a pathologcial state resulting from the reverse or impeded flow of blood in the body or the stagnation of blood flow in local parts as well as abnormal blood outside of the vessles which remains in the body and fails to disperse. As soon as blood stasis is formed, it can further affect the circulation of blood and lead to new pathological changes, causing a variety of diseases and syndromes. So it is also one of pathogenic factors.

Blood stasis is formed in two ways. In one way, it results from the impeded circulation of blood causesd by deficiency of *qi*, stagnation of *qi*, blood-cold and blood-heat, etc. For instance, deficiency of *qi* results in weak circulation of blood, stagnation of *qi* results in impeded circulation of blood, blood-cold results in coagulation of blood, and blood-heat results in the viscousness of blood. All these may impede the circulation of blood and cause blood stasis. In the other way, blood stasis is caused by abnormal blood outside of the vessels due to trauma or other reasons which fails to disperse and remains in the body.

核、瘰疬。

饮邪由于停留的部位不同而表现各异。如《金匮要略》说：“其人素盛今瘦，水走肠间，沥沥有声，谓之痰饮（狭义）；饮后水流胁下，咳唾引痛，谓之悬饮；饮水流行，归于四肢，当汗出而不汗出，身体疼痛，谓之溢饮；咳逆倚息，短气不得卧，其形如肿，谓之支饮。”

2. 瘀血

瘀血是指全身血脉运行不畅，或局部血行阻滞，以及体内有离经之血未能消散等病理状况。瘀血一旦形成，又可进一步影响气血运行，导致新的病理变化，形成多种病证，故亦属致病因素之一。

瘀血的形成，一是由于气虚、气滞、血寒、血热等原因，使血行不畅所致。如气虚则运血无力，气滞则血行不畅，血寒则血液凝滞，血热则血液粘滞，都可导致血行不畅而形成瘀血。二是因外伤及其他原因造成离经之血，未能消散，停留体内，而形成瘀血。

Blood stasis has different clinical manifestations in accordance with its stagnation in different parts of the body and the various reasons for its formations. For instance, blood stasis in the heart-vessels may lead to palpitation, chest tightness and precordial pain; stasis in the lung may lead to chest pain, cough with dyspnea and hemoptysis; stasis in the stomach may lead to stabbing pain in the stomach and tarry stool: stasis in the liver may lead to costalgia and hepatomegaly; invasion of blood stasis to the heart may lead to mania; stasis in the uterus may lead to pain in the lower abdomen, dysmenorrhea, amenorrhea, purplish red black and lumpy menstruation, or metrorrhagia and metrostaxis; stagnation of blood stasis in the terminal of the blood vessels of the extremities may lead to gangrene of finger and toe; stagnation of blood stasis in the local parts may cause loacl sweeling, pain and cyanosis.

Though diseases caused by blood stasis are many and diverse, their clinical manifestations can be summed up as follows: stabbing pain, cyanosis, tumour, bleeding (dark purplish blood with blood clots), dark complexion, squamous and dry skin, purplish dark tongue or with petechiae, ecchymosis, thready and uneven pulse, knotted pulse or intermittent pulse.

瘀血因其停留部位不同、形成原因各异，而有不同的临床表现。如瘀阻心脉，可见心悸、胸闷、心痛；瘀阻于肺,则见胸痛、咳喘、咯血；瘀阻于胃，可有胃脘刺痛、大便色黑；瘀阻于肝，可患胁痛、肝大；瘀血攻心，可致发狂；瘀阻胞宫，可有少腹疼痛、痛经、经闭、经色紫黑有块或崩漏；瘀血滞于肢体血脉末端，可致脱骨疽；瘀血阻于局部，可出现局部肿痛、青紫。

瘀血所致的病证虽较繁杂,但其临床表现可归纳为以下几点：即刺痛，紫绀，肿块，出血(血色紫暗并有血块)，面色黧黑，肌肤甲错，舌质紫暗或有瘀点、瘀斑，脉细涩或结代。

Chapter Two

PATHOGENESIS

Pathogenesis is the mechanism of the occurrence, development and change of a disease. It includes the pathogenic mechanism and the basic pathogenesis, which then can be interpreted respectively as follows.

Section 1

Pathogenic Mechanism

TCM regards the occurrence of a disease from the following two aspects: the deficiency of the vital-*qi* or the dysfunction of the human body; the pathological damage to the body. The so-called vital-*qi* refers to the normal physiological function of the body as well as its resistant and recovering capacity. It can be briefly called "*zheng*" in TCM. The so-called pathogenic factors widely refer to every kind of pathogenic element that leads to the occurrence of a disease. They are simply called "*xie*" in TCM.

1. The Deficiency of the Vital-*qi* Is the Internal Basic Cause of the Occurrence of a Disease

TCM focuses its attention on the vital-*qi* and holds that pathogenic factors can not invade the body so easily and cause a disease if the vital-*qi* is exuberant. According to the Chapter "Discussion on Acupuncture Methods" (Chapter 12), in

第 二 章

病 机

病机是疾病发生、发展与变化的机理，包括发病原理和基本病机两方面。现分述如下：

第一节 发病原理

中医学认为，疾病的发生有两方面的原因：一是人体正气不足或功能紊乱；二是邪气对人体的病理性损害。所谓正气，是指人体的正常生理功能及其抗病、康复能力，简称"正"；所谓邪气，乃泛指导致人体发病的各种致病因素，简称为"邪"。

1. 正气不足是发病的内在根据

中医学十分重视人体的正气，认为人体正气旺盛，邪气则难以侵入，疾病就不会发生。如《素问遗篇·刺法论》说："正气存内，

Plain Questions "Pathogenic factors can not cause trouble if the vital-*qi* is sufficient." Only when the vital-*qi* is comparatively insufficient and unable to defeat pathogenic factors, will the latter take the advantage of the body and attack it. Such phenomenon has been described in the Chapter "Discussion of Four Kinds of Febrile Diseases" (Chapter 33) in *Plain Questions*: "Where pathogenic factors accumulate, the parts of the body must be deficient in the vital-*qi*."

2. The Invasion of Pathogenic Factors Is the External Cause of the Occurrence of a Disease

TCM attaches great importance to the vital-*qi*. However, it does not exclude pathogenic factors, which actually function a great deal in causing a disease and even play a decisive role in some particular cases. For instance, in such cases as trauma, poisoning or snakebite, even if the vital-*qi* is exuberant, the victim will be hurt unavoidably and fall ill.

In a word, etiology of TCM believes that the occurrence of a disease is mainly involved in two aspects, namely, the vital-*qi* and pathogenic factors. And the deficiency of the vital-*qi* is considered to be the basic internal cause while the invasion of pathogenic factors as the important external cause of the occurrence of a disease.

Section 2

Basic Pathogenesis

In the course of a disease, various syndromes result from the different patients' constitution and invading factors. However, each syndrome has its own concrete patho-

邪不可干"。只有在正气相对不足，卫外不固时，邪气才会侵入人体而发病，即《素问·评热病论》所说："邪之所凑，其气必虚。"

2．邪气侵袭是发病的重要条件

中医学重视正气，并不排除邪气在发病中的重要作用。邪气是发病的条件，在某些特殊情况下，甚至起决定性作用。如外伤、中毒、毒蛇咬伤等，即使正气旺盛，亦难免被伤害而发病。

综上所述，中医发病学认为，疾病的发生是由正气与邪气两方面决定的：正气不足是发病的内在根据，邪气入侵是发病的重要条件。

第二节 基本病机

在疾病过程中，由于患者的体质不同，病邪各异，因而产生了各种不同的病证。而每一病证本身，都有其具体的病机变化。但

genesis. By and large, the basic pathogenesis is no more than the conflict between the vital-*qi* and pathogenic factors, the imbalance of *yin* and *yang* as well as the disturbance in ascending and descending of *qi*.

1. Conflict between *"Zheng"* and *"Xie"*

This refers to the conflict between the vital-*qi* and pathogenic factors. Such conflict is not only related closely to the occurrence of a disease but also affects the development and the final outcome of a disease. Meanwhile, it has some direct influence on the sthenic or asthenic transformation of a disease. Therefore, the course of a disease, in a sense, is that of the conflict between the vital-*qi* and pathogenic factors.

1) The Relation between the Conflict and the Transformation of the Deficiency or Excess

During the conflict, the vital-*qi* and pathogenic factors can influence each other and mutually wax and wane. Generally speaking, when the vital-*qi* is exuberant, it can suppress pathogenic factors so as to prevent a disease. However, either the deficiency of the vital-*qi* or the excess of pathogenic factors can lead to the failure of the vital-*qi* in conquering pathogenic factors. In such cases, pathogenic factors will take the advantage of the vital-*qi* and cause a disease. With the rise and fall of the conflict between the vital-*qi* and pathogenic factors, the transformation of syndromes from the deficiency to the excess and vice versa appear.

According to the Chapter "General Discussion on Sthenia and Asthenia"(Chapter 28) in *Plain Questions,*"Excess syndrome results when the invading pathogens are exuberant while exhaustion of the vital essence brings on deficiency syndrome." Excess syndrome mainly indicates the excess of pathogenic factors, namely, the pathological development mostly based on the excess of pathogenic factors. In such cases, pathogenic factors are excessive while the patient's vital-*qi* is strong enough to resist

从总体上来说，基本病机不外正邪斗争、阴阳失调和升降失常三方面。

2. 正邪斗争

正邪斗争是指正气与病邪的斗争。这种斗争不仅关系着疾病的发生，而且影响着疾病的发展与转归，同时也直接影响着病证的虚实变化。因此，从某种意义上讲，许多疾病的过程，就是正邪斗争的过程。

1) 正邪斗争与虚实变化　正邪双方在斗争过程中是互为消长的。一般说来，若正气强盛，正能胜邪，人体就不会发病。若正气虚弱，或邪气偏盛，均可导致正不胜邪，出现邪胜正负而发生疾病。随着正邪斗争的消长、盛衰，形成了病证的虚实变化。

《素问·通评虚实论》说："邪气盛则实，精气夺则虚。" 实，主要是指邪气亢盛，即以邪气亢盛为主要方面的病理变化。其病理特点是：邪气亢盛而正气未衰，正气足以与邪气抗争，故正邪斗

pathogenic factors at the same time, thus the conflict between the two sides is very intense, which clinically shows excess syndrome of strong reaction. Such syndrome can be found in the early or middle stage of exopathic diseases or those diseases due to the stagnation of phlegm, food, water and blood within the human body. The symptoms like high fever, mania, loud speaking and coarse breathing, abdominal pain with tenderness, uroschesis and constipation, replete pulse, belong to excess syndrome.

Deficiency mainly refers to the kind of pathological change with the insufficiency of the vital-qi as its leading aspect. Its pathological features are: the vital-qi is too weak to resist pathogenic factors, so the pathological reaction is less intense. Clinically, the patient tends to be weak in terms of the vital-qi. The deficiency syndrome is mostly found in such cases as weak constitution or later stage of a disease and various kinds of chronic diseases. Its clinical manifestations are lassitude and sallow complexion, palpitation and short breath, spontaneous perspiration, night sweat or dysphoria with feverish sensation in the chest, palms and soles, or cold limbs and feeble pulse.

The conflict between the vital-qi and pathogenic factors can not only produce such effects as pure excess syndrome or deficiency syndrome, but also lead to the coexistance of deficiency syndrome and excess syndrome. Among them, the deficiency intermingled with excess condition refers to the deficiency syndrome complicated with excess syndrome while the former is dominant, which can be found in the patient with dropsy due to insufficiency of the spleen and so on; as for the excess intermingled with some deficiency condition, it means excess syndrome dominates with some manifestations of deficiency, such as the case of consumption of body fluid due to excessive heat. For the same reason, the disease can turn from excess to deficiency and vice versa since the conflicting sides are frequently interchangable.

争激烈，临床表现为反应剧烈的实证。实证多见于外感病的初、中期，或由痰、食、水、血等滞留体内所引起的病证，如壮热、狂躁、声高气粗、腹痛拒按、二便不通、脉实有力等。

虚，主要是指正气不足，即以正气虚损为主要方面的病理变化。其病理特点是：正气已虚，无力与邪抗争，病理反应不剧烈，临床可出现一系列虚弱、无力和不足的证候。虚证多见于素体虚弱病人或疾病后期以及多种慢性病，临床表现为神疲乏力、面容憔悴、心悸气短、自汗、盗汗或五心烦热，或畏寒肢冷、脉虚无力等。

正邪斗争的消长、盛衰不仅可以产生单纯的虚证、实证，而且在复杂的疾病中，因治疗不当或失治，导致正气已伤，而邪气久留；或因正气本虚，无力驱邪；或正气不足，内生水湿、痰饮、瘀血等，形成虚中挟实、实中挟虚的虚实错杂证候。其中，虚中挟实是指以正虚为主、又挟实邪的病证，如脾虚水肿；实中挟虚则是指以邪实为主、又兼见虚候的病证，如热盛伤津。由于邪正双方斗争力量的对比经常发生变化，因此疾病亦可由实转虚或由虚转实。

It is necessary to point out that usually the phenomenon and nature of a disease are consistent with each other, thus manifesting excess syndrome or deficiency syndrome of pathogenesis correspondingly. However, under some particular circumstances, the opposite situation will occur, hence the "appearance of deficiency in extreme excess" (i.e. excess in reality with pseudo-deficiency symptoms) and "symptoms of excess in extreme deficiency" (i.e. deficiency in reality with pseudo-excess symptoms). These two phenomena have to be carefully distinguished clinically.

2) **The Relation between the Conflict and the Final Outcome of a Disease**

In the course of a disease, the conflict between the vital-*qi* and pathogenic factors not only shows up the deficiency or excess of a disease, but also deteimines the outcome of the disease. If the vital-*qi* prevails, the disease takes a favourable turn or recovers completely; if pathogenic factors prevail, the disease takes an unfavourable turn or even deteriorates and may result in death then.

The most common outcome of many diseases lies in the dominant position of the vital-*qi*. If the patient has fairly excessive vital-*qi*, resulting in considerable capability to resist pathogenic factors, or he has been given the prompt and proper treatment, then pathological factors are restrained in development, correspondingly, their pathogenic actions are weakening or disappear; the functions of pathologically damaged viscera, channels and collaterals, tissues as well as organs will progressively recover; the consumptions of essence of life, the vital-*qi*, blood and body fluid will gradually be remedied; *yin* and *yang* will regain their relative balance on the new basis and finally the disease is cured.

The domination of pathogenic factors over the vital-*qi* results when a disease turns towards deterioration or even death. If the vital-*qi* is too weak or pathogenic factors are too strong,

需要指出的是，在一般情况下，疾病的现象与本质是相符的，能够反映病机的虚与实。但在某些特殊情况下，会出现疾病的现象与本质相反的情况，如"大实有羸状（即真实假虚）"和"至虚有盛候（即真虚假实）"。临床时应注意鉴别。

　　2）正邪斗争与疾病转归　在疾病过程中，正邪双方的斗争不仅反映出疾病的虚与实，而且决定着疾病的转归。正胜邪退，则疾病趋向好转或痊愈；邪胜正衰，则疾病趋向加重或恶化，甚至导致死亡。

　　正胜邪退是许多疾病最常见的一种转归。如果患者正气比较充盛，抗御病邪的能力较强，或因得到了及时而正确的治疗，邪气就难以进一步发展，对机体的毒害作用减弱或消失，脏腑、经络、组织、器官的病理损害逐渐得到修复，精、气、血、津液等的耗伤也逐渐得到恢复，机体阴阳两方面在新的基础上又获得动态平衡，疾病即可痊愈。

　　邪胜正衰是疾病向恶化甚至死亡方面转归的一种结局。如果

the capability of the organism to resist pathogenic factors becomes weaker gradually and is unable to restratin the development of pathogenic factors, then the pathological damage to the organism increasingly becomes more severe and the disease will deteriorate each day. If the vital-qi exhausts while pathogenic factors dominate, then the functions of viscera, ehannels and collaterals become weakened; the essence of life, vital-qi, blood and body fluid are exhausted; yin and $yang$ will depart forever and life comes to an end.

Besides, in the course of a disease, it may turn up that the vital-qi is deficient with pathogenic factors still clinging to the body or pathogenic factors are already removed and the vital-qi is still deficient. As a result, the disease gets prolongated and lasts uncured, thus turning from acute to chronic or having some sequelae left.

2. Imbalance of *Yin* and *Ying*

The imbalance of *yin* and *yang* refers to the pathological state of the organism in which the two sides lose their balance and coordination under the influence of pathological factors. Since the viscera, channels and collaterals, qi, blood, *ying* and *wei*, the inward and outward, ascending and descending motion of qi in the human body can be divided into *yin* and *yang*, the various kinds of pathogenic factors such as six exogenous factors, seven emotions, improper diet and overfatigue can only form a disease by way of the imbalance of *yin* and *yang* of the organism, so the imbalance of *yin* and *yang* is a high summary of various kinds of pathogenesis relating to losing balance, and is also the most basic pathogenesis of all kinds of pathological changes. Although the pathological change of the imbalance of *yin* and *yang* is very complicated, its manifestations are no more than the following aspects:

1) Relative Excess of *Yin* or *Yang*

It mainly refers to the fact that „the excess syndrome results

正气虚弱或邪气太盛，机体抗病能力日趋低下，不能制止邪气的发展，机体受到的病理性损害逐渐加重，病情就会趋向恶化。若正气衰竭，邪气独盛，脏腑、经络功能衰惫，精、气、血、津液枯竭，甚至阴阳离决，生命活动亦告终止而死亡。

此外，在疾病过程中，也可出现正虚邪恋或邪去而正虚的情况，则易使病程延长，日久不愈，疾病由急性转为慢性，或留下某些后遗症。

2．阴阳失调

阴阳失调，是指机体在致病因素作用下所发生的阴阳双方失去协调、平衡的病理状态。由于人体的脏腑、经络、气血、营卫以及气机的升降出入等皆有阴阳之分，六淫、七情、饮食、劳倦等各种致病因素，必须通过导致机体内部的阴阳失调才能形成疾病。所以阴阳失调是对人体各种失去平衡协调病机的高度概括，也是人体各种病变的最基本病机。尽管阴阳失调的病理变化十分复杂，但其表现形式不外以下几个方面：

1）阴阳偏胜　阴或阳偏胜主要是指"邪气盛则实"的实证。

when the invading pathogens is exuberant." Pathogenic factors tend to go in accordance with the categorical characteristics when they invade the human body. Namely, when *yang* pathogen sets in, it will cause the excess of *yang;* and when *yin* pathogen intrudes, it will cause the excess of *yin*.

The excess of *yang* suggests a pathological state in which *yang* is excessive and the organism is in a hyperfunctional condition. Its pathological feature is the excessive *yang* with inapparent deficiency of *yin*. The excess of *yang* is mostly due to warm or heat pathogens as well as the transformation from infected *yin* pathogen to *yang* and heat; or the internal damage caused by the upset of seven emotions, such as the fire syndromes caused by the overaction of five emotions or the stagnated *qi*, blood stasis, indigestion and some others. *Yang* is featured with heat, motion and driness, so the manifestations of *yang* excess are mainly high fever, aversion to heat, restlessness, red tongue, dry, rough and yellowish fur, or abdominal distention and pain with tenderness, tidal fever, delirium and so on.

Since the excess of *yang* can lead to disorder of *yin*, it can also be accompanied by *yin* deficiency with the symptoms of thirsy, desiring for cold drink, constipation, oliguria and so on.

The excess of *yin* means the pathological state in which *yin* is excessive, the function of the organism declines and the pathological products accumulate in the course of a disease. Its pathological feature is the excess *yin* with the inapparent deficiency of *yang*. The excess of *yin* is mainly due to the infected cold dampness and other *yin* pathogens, overating something raw or cold, or the stagnation and obstruction with pathogenic cold inside so that *yang* is unable to limit *yin*, which leads to the consequent excess of *yin*-coldness. *Yin* is featured with coldness, quietness and dampness, thus the manifestations of the excess of *yin* are mainly aversion to cold, quietness, epigastric pain with tenderness, loose stool and so on.

Since the excess of *yin* can lead to the disorder of *yang*, it

病邪侵入人体必从其类，即阳邪侵入人体可形成阳偏胜；阴邪侵入人体则形成阴偏胜。

阳偏胜，是指机体在疾病过程中所出现的阳气偏胜、机能亢进的病理状态。其病理特点是阳虽盛但阴虚不明显。阳偏胜形成的原因主要是由于感受温热阳邪；或虽感受阴邪，但从阳化热；或七情内伤，五志过极化火，以及气滞、血瘀、食积等郁而化火所致。阳以热、动、燥为特点，故阳偏胜多表现为壮热、恶热、烦躁不安、舌红、苔黄燥，或腹部胀满、腹痛拒按、潮热、谵语等实热证。

由于阳胜则阴病，故阳偏胜还可兼见口渴、喜凉饮、大便秘结、小便短少等阴亏症状。

阴偏胜，是指机体在疾病过程中所出现的阴气偏胜、机能衰退以及病理产物积聚的病理状态。其病理特点是阴虽盛但阳虚不明显。阴偏胜的形成原因主要是由于感受寒湿阴邪，或过食生冷，寒滞中阻，因而阳不制阴，阴寒内盛。阴以寒、静、湿为特点，故阴偏胜多表现为恶寒、沉静、脘腹冷痛拒按、大便溏泄等寒实证。

由于阴胜则阳病，故阴偏胜还可兼见形寒肢冷、神疲踡卧等

can also have such manifestations as chilly appearance and cold limbs, lassitude with the inclination to stay in bed with flexion of legs and so on.

2) **Relative Deficiency of** *Yin* **or** *Yang*

This refers to the deficient syndrome that "exhaustion of vital essence brings on deficiency syndrome."

The deficiency of *yang* suggests such a pathological state in which *yang-qi* is insuffcient, the function of the organism declines and warmness is lacked in the course of a disease. Its pathological features are the scarcity of *yang*, the failure of *yang* in limiting *yin* and the relative excess of *yin*. The deficiency of *yang* is mostly in conseuqence of the congenital defect or improper care after birth, or the over-fatigue or persisting disease leading to the chronic damage of *yang*. The deficiency of *yang* will produce the effect of cold syndrome, so clinically its symptoms are mostly chill and cold limbs, lassitude with the inclination to stay in bed with flexion of legs, abdominal pain alleviated by warmness and pressure, loose stool, copious and clear urine, slow and feeble pulse, etc.

The deficiency of *yin*, namely the weakness of *yin*, indicates the pathological state as which the *yin*-fluid is too weak to check *yang*, manifested as weak hyperfunction. It is featured with the insufficiency of *yin*-fluid, attenuation of the functions of nourishing, quietening and conditioning *yang*-heat, *yang* is relatively excessive and there appears the heat syndrome of deficiency type. The deficiency of *yin* is mostly in the consequence of pathogenic damage from *yang* extending to *yin*, or syndromes caused by the overatcion of five emotions and five transmissions leading to the impairment of *yin*, or the damage of *yin*-fluid due to chronic diseases, or the injury of *yin* caused by overeating dry and hot foods. The deficiency of *yin* will consequently produce heat syndromes of deficiency type, manifested as dysphoria with feverish sensation in the chest, palms and soles, hectic fever, flushed face, emaciation, night sweat, dry throat

阳虚症状。

2) 阴阳偏衰 阴或阳偏衰，是指"精气夺则虚"的虚证。

阳偏衰，即阳虚，是指机体在疾病过程中所出现的阳气虚损、机能减退、温煦不足的病理状态。其病理特点是阳气不足，阳不制阴，阴相对亢盛。阳偏衰多因先天禀赋不足，或后天失养或劳倦内伤，以及久病损伤阳气所致。阳虚则寒，故临床多表现为畏寒肢冷、神疲踡卧、腹痛喜温喜按、大便稀溏、小便清长、脉迟无力等虚寒证。

阴偏衰，即阴虚，是机体在疾病过程中所出现的阴液不足，不能制阳，机能虚性兴奋的病理状态。其病理特点是阴液不足，其滋养、宁静和制约阳热的功能减退，阳气相对亢奋，出现虚热证。阴偏衰多因阳邪伤阴，或五志过极化火伤阴，或久病耗伤阴液，或过食燥热之物伤阴所致。阴虚则热，故临床多表现为五心烦热、骨蒸潮热、面红升火、消瘦、盗汗、咽干口燥、舌红少苔、脉细

and thirst, red tongue with thin coating, thready and rapid pulse.

3) **Mutual Damage of** *Yin* **nad** *Yang*

This suggests the pathogenesis of the deficiency of both *yin* and *yang* due to the pathological change of either side with secondary involvement of the other.

Yin damage extends to *yang* when the deficiency of *yin* has reached such an extent that *yang-qi* is involved, so that the production of *yang* is insufficient or exhausts because of the detachment, thus developing into a pathological state in which *yin* deficiency and *yang* deficiency coexist but *yin* deficiency dominates. For instance, dizziness and lassitude in loins and knees due to the deficiency of kindey-*yin* once involve the kidney-*yang's* production, the symptoms like impotence, cold limbs, will occur.

Yang damage extends to *yin* when the deficiency of *yang* is serious enough to interfere with the production of *yin* fluid, so that such a pathological state appears in which both *yin* and *yang* are deficient with the domination of *yang*. Take for example the edema due to insufficiency of *yang*, once it gains the chance to influence the production of *yin*-essence, the symptoms such as emaciation, vexation, or even clonic convulsion, may occur.

4) **Repellence between** *Yin* **and** *Yang*

This refers to such a pathological state in which either *yin* or *yang* is extremely excessive, and stagnated and choked inside, or either *yin* or *yang* is too deficient so that the powers of the two sides are of great disparity. The stronger one will repel the weaker one. As a result, *yin* and *yang* are separated. Syndromes such as cold syndrome with pseudo-heat symptoms or heat syndrome with pseudo-cold symptoms will occur.

The excessive *yin* will repel *yang*. This refers to such a pathological state in which *yang* is too deficient to check *yin*, the excessive cold pathogens will be stagnated inside the body and repel *yang-qi* to the exterior, *yin* and *yang* are separated. According to Clause No. 317 of *Treatise on Febrile Diseases:* "*Shaoyin* syndrome with diarrhea, interior cold with heat outside,

数等虚热证。

3）阴阳互损　阴阳互损，是指在阴或阳任何--方虚损到相当程度，病变又累及其相对的一方，造成阴阳两虚的病理状态。

阴损及阳，是指阴虚到相当程度，又累及阳的一方，使阳气化生不足或无所依附而耗散，从而形成以阴虚为主、阴阳两虚的病理状态。如肾阴不足，出现头晕目眩、腰膝酸软，一旦累及肾阳的化生，可同时兼见阳萎、肢冷等肾阳虚的症状。

阳损及阴，是阳虚较重又累及阴液的化生，使阴液生成不足，从而形成以阳虚为主、阴阳两虚的病理状态。如阳虚水泛的水肿，一旦累及阴精的生成，可同时兼见消瘦、心烦、甚至瘛疭等阴虚症状。

4）阴阳格拒　阴阳格拒，是阴或阳某一方偏胜至极，壅遏于内；或一方极端虚弱，双方盛衰悬殊，盛者踞于内，将另一方排斥、格拒于外，使阴阳之间不相维系，出现真寒假热或真热假寒等复杂的病理现象。

阴盛格阳，是指阳气极度虚弱，阳不制阴，阴寒之邪壅盛于内，逼迫阳气浮越于外，阴阳气不相维系，相互格拒的病理状态。

cold extremities, barely palpable pulse, flushed complexion without aversion to cold ...". This can be one of the examples of excessive *yin* with *yang* repelled outside.

The excessive *yang* will repel *yin*. This means that when the pathogenic heat is strong and hidden deeply in the human body, *yang* is kept chocked in the interior and unable to reach the four limbs, *yin* is rejected outside. According to Clause No. 350 of **Treatise on Febrile Diseases**: "A patient of exogenous febrile disease with cold limbs and slippery pulse due to internal heat can be cured with White Tiger Decoction which functions in clearing out the interior heat." This is one of the examples of excessive *yang* with *yin* repelled outside.

5) **Exhaustion of** *Yin* **and** *Yang*

It includes the exhaustion of either *yin* or *yang*. It suggests such a pathological state in which *yin*-fluid or *yang*-qi is suddenly exhausted in a great deal so that the state of impending death appears.

The exhaustion of *yang* refers to such a pathological state in which the sudden serious exhaustion of *yang*-qi causes the danger of life. Generally speaking, the exhaustion of *yang* is mainly due to excessive pathogenic factors which are beyond the vital-*qi*'s capacity to resist; or the constitution of *yang* asthenia, deficiency of the vital-*qi* and the extravagantly-consumed *qi* caused by overstrain; it is also likely to be the result of overuse of diaphoretic, emetic, or purgative therapy, or the excess of sweat, vomiting and purgation so that *yang* has been exhausted with body fluid, or to be the consequence of the extreme deficiency of *yang* in chronic diseases which have made *yang* stay outside. Clinically, its manifestations are mostly profuse sweating, cold extremeties and skin, lassitude, apathy or even coma, faint pulse, etc.

The exhaustion of *yin* refers to such a pathological state in which the sudden exhaustion of the *yin*-fluid leads to the serious declination of the systematic functions of the whole body. Usual-

如《伤寒论》317条所说"少阴下利，里寒外热，手足厥逆，脉微欲绝，身反不恶寒，其人面色赤"，即为例证。

阳盛格阴，是指邪热极盛，阳热之邪深伏于里，阳气被遏，不能外达四肢，而格阴于外的病理状态。如《伤寒论》350条所说"伤寒，脉滑而厥者，里有热，白虎汤主之"，即为例证。

5) 阴阳亡失　包括亡阴、亡阳两大类，是指机体的阴液或阳气突然大量地亡失，导致生命垂危的病理状态。

亡阳，是指人体阳气突然发生严重衰竭，而致生命垂危的病理状态。一般说来，亡阳多因邪气过盛，正不敌邪；或素体阳虚，正气不足，疲劳过度，耗气过甚；或误用汗、吐、下等法，或汗、吐、下过度，阳随津泄；或久病阳气极虚等，使虚阳外越所致。其临床表现多为大汗淋漓、肌肤手足厥冷、精神疲惫、表情淡漠，甚至昏迷、脉微欲绝等。

亡阴，是指人体阴液发生突然性消耗或脱失，而致全身机能严重衰竭的另一病理状态。一般说来，亡阴多因邪热炽盛，或邪

ly, the exhaustion of *yin* is chiefly due to the excess of pathogenic heat, t' e persistance of pathogenic heat which has wasted *yin*-fluid in great amounts, or the extreme damage to *yin*-fluid caused by improper treatment and some other factors. Clinically, the manifestions are continuous sweating, hot greasy sweating, warm limbs, thirsty and desiring for cold drinks, wrinkled skin, deep hollowed eyes, restlessness or coma, rapid and thready pulse, or large and weak pulse.

Since *yin* and *yang* depend on each other, the exhaustion of *yin* will check the production of *yang* and vice versa. Correspondingly, the exhaustion of *yin* will soon lead to the exhaustion of *yang;* and the exhaustion of *yang* will influence *yin* in the same way. Therefore, either the exhaustion of *yin* or that of *yang* can finally lead to the separation of the two sides with the ensuing of death although they may have different pathogenesis and various manifestations.

3. Disturbance of Ascending and Descending

This widely refers to such a pathological state in which the ascending or descending movement of the viscera's functional activities are disordered and *yin*, *yang*, *qi*, blood are imbalanced under the influence of pathogenic factors.

Since the ascending and descending, inletting and outletting movements of the functional activities closely relate to various aspects of the viscera, channels and collaterals, *qi* and blood, *yin* and *yang*, their disturbance may cause the functional abnormality of five *zang*-organs, six *fu*-organs, the interior and exterior, four limbs and nine orifices: the flaring-up of heart-fire will lead to aphthous stomatitis; the impairment of dispersion and descending function of the lung will lead to cough, asthma and oppressed feeling in the chest; the impaired ascending function of the spleen will lead to the result of loose stool; the upward inversion of the liver-*qi* will lead to the result of vertigo, and distention in head; the failure of receiving *qi*

热久留,大量煎灼阴液,或因误治等其他因素大量损耗阴液所致。其临床表现多为汗出不止,汗热而粘,四肢温和,渴喜冷饮,皮肤皱摺,眼窝深陷,烦躁或昏迷,脉细数无力或大而无力等。

亡阴、亡阳虽病机不同,表现各异,但由于阴阳互根,阴亡则阳无以生,阳亡则阴无以化,故亡阴可迅速导致亡阳,亡阳亦可继而出现亡阴,最终均可导致"阴阳离决"而死亡。

3. 升降失常

升降失常,泛指在致病因素作用下,导致脏腑气机升降出入运动紊乱、阴阳气血失调的病理状态。

由于气机的升降出入关系到脏腑、经络、气血、阴阳等各个方面,故升降出入失常可导致五脏六腑、表里内外、四肢九窍等各组织、器官功能异常。如心火上炎,则口舌生疮;肺失宣降,则咳喘、胸闷;脾不升清,则大便溏泄;肝气上逆,则眩晕、头胀;

in the kidney will lead to the prolonged expiration and shortened inspiration as well as short breath. The normal condition of the six-*fu*-organs is measured with their smooth movements of descending. If the gallbladder-*qi* goes up, it will result in vomiting of bilious fluid; if the stomach-*qi* fails to descend, it will result in nausea, vomiting, hiccup, belching; the disorder of the large intestine's transportation may lead to abdominal distention and constipation; the dysfunction of the urinary bladder may result in dysuria or even uroschesis. When the ascending adverseness of *yin, yang, qi* and blood obstructs the brain, syncope and unconsciousness will occur.

TCM also expounds such a theory that the disturbance of the movements of ascending, descending, inletting and outletting manifests respective emphasis on both exopathic disease and internal injury. The pathogenesis of exopathic disease comes from outside, so the emphasis is on the imbalance between inletting and outletting; the pathogenesis of the internal injury comes from the inside, so the emphasis is laid on the imbalance between ascending and descending. Ascending and descending, inletting and outletting closely relate to each other not only in physiology but also in pathology. In the case of cough with dyspnea caused by wind-cold pathogen, the invasion of the superficial part of the body by wind-cold may cause both the muscular striae and the sweat gland to be shut up, and the defensive *qi* obstructed, the manifestations of which are aversion to cold, fever and anhidrosis caused by imbalance between inletting and outletting. Since the lung is related to the skin and hair, the superficial pathogen can not be repelled, and the lung is affected, thus leading to the conseuqence of impairment of dispersion and descending of the lung, the manifestations of which are cough and dyspnea resulting from the imbalance of ascending and descending. The two cases above are the examples of the mutual influence between the imbalance of inletting and outletting and that of ascending and descending.

肾不纳气，则呼多吸少、气短息促。六腑以通降为顺，若胆气上逆，则呕吐苦水；胃失和降，则恶心、呕吐、呃逆、嗳气；大肠传导失职，则腹胀、便秘；膀胱气化不行，则小便不利或尿闭。若阴阳气血逆乱并走于上蒙蔽清窍，则出现突然昏倒、不省人事等症状。

中医学认为，外感病与内伤病在升降出入失常方面，各有所偏重。外感病邪从外来，故以出入失常为主；内伤病邪自内生，故以升降失常为重。但升降与出入，在生理上密切相关，病理上亦互相影响。如外感风寒之咳喘证，风寒袭表，肌腠郁闭，汗孔闭塞，卫气不能宣通，症见恶寒、发热、无汗，是出入失常的表现；肺合皮毛，表邪不解，内舍于肺，肺失肃降，症见咳喘、气逆，又是升降失常的表现。此即出入失常与升降失常相互影响的例证。

脾胃为后天之本，居于中焦，通上连下，为升降出入运动的

The spleen and stomach provide material basis for the acquired constitution. They are in the middle part of the body, linking the upper and the lower part of the body so as to function as a pivot in the movements of ascending, descending, inletting and outletting. The coordination of the spleen and stomach's ascending and descending functions and the good order of their inletting and outletting movements may make the clear-*qi* ascend and the turbid-*qi* descend in order to nourish the whole body and expel the nuisance, and make the physiological functions of other internal organs work normally. The disorder of the ascending and descending movements of the spleen and stomach will involve the following abnormalities: the distribution of *yang-qi* is checked; the acquired essence can not be stored up; neither food and drinks nor oxygen can be taken in; the product of metabolism can not be expelled out and consequently the other internal organs may be affected. From the above mentioned abnormalities many diseases will arise. Thus TCM has been putting a great deal of emphasis on regulating the functions of the spleen and stomach.

枢纽。脾胃升降正常，出入有序，则能维持升清降浊、营养全身

和排泄糟粕的功能，并使其他脏腑的生理作用得以正常发挥。若

脾胃升降出入失常，则清阳之气不能敷布，后天之精不能归藏，

饮食、精气无法摄入，代谢废物不能排出，并可影响其他脏腑，

百病由之而生。故历代医家在治疗疾病时均十分重视调理脾胃的

功能。

Chapter Three
PREVENTION

Prevention is to take certain precautions against the occurrence and progress of a disease.

TCM has been through all the ages attaching great importance to prevention. As early as over two thousand years ago, the theory of "Preventive Treatment of a Disease" was put forward in the book *Yellow Emperor's Canon of Internal Medicine*. This theory, in fact, includes two aspects: adopting preventive measures before a disease comes and taking precautions against the progression of a disease.

Section 1
Taking Preventive Measures

It refers to taking various precautions against the possible occurrence of a disease. As mentioned above, the occurrence of a disease is due to both deficiency of the vital-*qi* and dysfunction of the human body and the pathological damages to the human body caused by pathogenic factors. Hence, the prevention of a disease should also start with these two aspects.

1. Building up the Vital-*qi*'s Power to Resist Pathogenic Factors

The fluctuation of the vital-*qi* depends primarily on one's constitution. Generally speaking, a man with strong constitution possesses sufficient vital-*qi* while a constitutionally feeble

第 三 章
预 防

预防，就是采取一定的措施，防止疾病发生和发展。

中医历来重视疾病的预防，早在两千多年前，《黄帝内经》中就已提出了"治未病"的预防思想。所谓"治未病"，实际上包括未病先防和既病防变两个方面的内容。

第一节 未 病 先 防

未病先防是指在未病之前，就做好各种预防工作，以防止疾病的发生。如前所述，疾病的发生，一是因人体正气不足或功能紊乱，二是因邪气对人体造成的病理损害。因此，预防疾病的发生亦应从这两方面来着手。

1. 增强正气的抗邪能力

人体正气的强弱，主要取决于人的体质。一般来说，体质强

man has deficient vital-*qi*. Accordingly, it is of crucial importance to strengthen the constitution in improving the resistence of the vital-*qi* to pathogenic factors. The physical condition of a person is mainly concerned with such aspects as innate factors, diet regulation, physical exercises and mental state, all of which should, therefore, be taken into consideration if one wants to be stronger.

1) Endorsing Eugenics

One inherits the innate factors from his parents. So, the parents' health status can directly influence the baby's constitution. Many kinds of diseases have something to do with genetic factors. TCM has also observed that "the majority of the children borne by underage parents are weak in constitution" (from *A Complete Work on Pediatrics*, by Chen Fuzheng, Qing Dynasty). Thereby, late marriage and eugenics should be advocated to ensure the children a sound constitution.

2) Leading a Regular Life

Living in nature, one should not only understand but also adapt himself to the changing patterns of the natural environment. Only proper control and arrangement of diet, daily life, work and rest can secure one with a strong body. According to the Chapter "Discussion on How to keep Innate Vitality *Qi*" (Chapter 1) in *Plain Questions*, "One, who knows the ways of health preservation, complies with natural law, adapts himself to the variations in nature, keeps a moderate diet, leads a regular life and shuns overwork, will obtain both physical and mental health which is the promise of longevity of over one hundred years." The book also persuades one not to "drink excessively, indulge himself in sexual pleasures, act willfully, exhaust all his energies, squander away his essence of life and spirit without any sense of preserving them, follow his aimless inclinations and lead a careless life with no enjoyment of a healthy life."

3) Doing More Physical Exercises

Frequent physical exercises can improve one's constitution,

者，正气盛；体质弱者，正气虚。因此，增强体质是提高正气抗邪能力的关键，而人的体质强弱主要与先天禀赋、饮食调养、身体锻炼和精神状态有关。因此，要增强体质，亦须从这几方面入手。

1) 优生优育 先天禀赋取决于父母。父母的健康状况，能直接影响子女的身体基本素质。不少疾病的发生，与遗传因素有关。中医还观察到"年少生子者，或多羸弱"（清·陈复正《幼幼集成》）。因此，应提倡晚婚和优生优育，以保证下一代有强壮的体质。

2) 生活应有规律 人生活在自然界，应该懂得并适应自然界的变化规律，对饮食、起居、劳逸等，都要有适当的节制和安排，即生活有规律，才能健康生长。如《素问·上古天真论》说："知其道者，法于阴阳，和于术数，饮食有节，起居有常，不妄作劳，故能形与神俱，而尽终其天年，度百岁乃去"。不可"以酒为浆，以妄为常，醉以入房，以欲竭其精，以耗散其真，不知持满，不时御神，务快其心，逆于生乐，起居无节。"

3) 加强锻炼 经常锻炼身体，能增强体质，提高正气的抗

strengthen the vital-qi to combat against pathogenic factors as well as to reduce or prevent the occurrence of diseases. The functions of accelerating the circulation of blood and qi, promoting the nimbleness of joints and keeping in good order the function and activities of qi can all be found in such physical exercises as the "Five-Mimic-Animal Boxing" created by Doctor Hua Tuo of Han Dynasty, the "Illustration of Physical and Breathing Exercises" copied on silk excavated from a grave of the Han Dynasty in Changsha, as well as those developed in later ages, such as *Taiji* Boxing, *Baduan Jin*, *Yijin Jing* and Chinese *Qigong*. All these exercises can be done to build up one's constitution and prevent diseases.

4) **Promoting Mental Health**

The mental activities of man are closely related to his physiological and pathological changes. It means a great deal in prevention and treatment of a disease to keep high spirits and stable mental state, and try one's best to avoid or reduce harmful mental stimulation or over-excitement. According to Chapter 1 of *Plain Questions*, "How can a disease occur if one keeps a serene mind, rejects lust and vain hope, keeps the vitality qi in a good condition and maintains a sound mind ?"

5) **Preventing Diseases with Traditional Chinese Drugs**

The Chapter "Discussion on Acupuncture Therapy" in (Chapter 72) *Plain Questions* says: "The pills of *Xiaojing Dan* will keep epidemic diseases away." This proves that prevention with traditional Chinese drugs has been practised for a long time in China. In recent years, TCM has been making wide use of the Chinese medicinal herbs for disease prevention. Satisfactory effects have been obtained in prevention of bacillary dysentry with garlic and portualca oleracea, of virus hepatitis with oriental wormwood, capejasmine and Chinese-date, and of influenza with isatis leaf and isatis root.

6) **Providing Artificial Immunity**

邪能力，减少或防止疾病的发生。如汉代医学家华佗创造的"五禽戏"，长沙汉墓出土的帛书《导引图》，以及后世的太极拳、八段锦、易筋经和气功等多种健身方法，均有促进血脉流通、关节滑利和气机调畅的作用，可用以增强体质，防治疾病。

4）调养精神　人的精神活动与机体的生理、病理变化密切相关。保持精神愉快、情绪安定，尽量避免或减少不良的精神刺激或过度的情绪波动，对防病、治病都具有重要意义。如《素问·上古天真论》说："恬憺虚无，真气从之，精神内守，病安从来。"

5）中药预防　《素问遗篇·刺法论》说："小金丹……服十粒，无疫干也。"说明中国在很早以前就开始采用中药预防疾病。近几年来，中国医务人员广泛采用中草药预防疾病，如用大蒜、马齿苋预防菌痢，用茵陈、栀子、大枣预防病毒性肝炎，用大青叶、板蓝根预防流感等，都取得了较好的效果。

6）人工免疫　早在十六世纪，中国就发明了人痘接种预防

In the sixteenth century, the Chinese invented variolation to prevent smallpox, which has crowned them as the forerunner of the world in the field of immunology. Modern Chinese doctors have combined traditional Chinese medicine with modern immunological techniques to prevent diseases with the result of the eradication of such fulminating infections as smallpox and the plague as well as the effective control of some other communicable diseases.

2. Taking Precautions against the Invasion of Pathogenic Factors

Pathogenic factors play an important or, sometimes, even decisive role in disease-causing. So, the preventive treatment of diseases means not only the improvement of constitution and the strengthening of the vital-*qi* against pathogenic factors, but also the prevention of the invasion by pathogenic factors. According to Chapter 1 of *Plain Questions*, "Pathogenic factors, especially pathogenic wind, are harmful and should be guarded against at all times." This means that people should do their utmost to avoid the invasion of six exogenous factors and pestilence. A chapter of *Synopsis of Prescriptions of the Golden Chamber*, "the Treatise on Indications and Contraindications of Fowls, Animals, Fish and Worms" tells us that "Dirty food, rotten meat and stinking fish are harmful to people. The six kinds of animals, whenever they die of themselves, die of pestilence. So, they are poisonous and can not be taken as food." Therefore, people should pay much attention to food hygiene. As for trauma, it can be avoided if safety precaution are taken in work and daily life.

Section 2
Preventing the Progression of a Disease

It is ideal to prevent the disease before it attacks a body.

天花，可谓世界免疫学的先驱。近代，中国医务人员除采用传统中医方法预防疾病外，还积极采用现代免疫学技术预防疾病，从而消灭了天花、鼠疫等烈性传染病，并使其他传染病也得到了有效的控制。

2．防止病邪的侵害

病邪是导致疾病发生的重要条件，有时甚至起决定性作用。故治未病除了增强体质，提高正气的抗邪能力外，还应注意防止病邪的侵害。如《素问·上古天真论》说："虚邪贼风，避之有时"，是说应尽量避免六淫、疫疠的侵袭。《金匮要略·禽兽鱼虫禁忌并治》说："秽饭、馁肉、臭鱼，食之伤人。……六畜自死，皆疫死，则有毒，不可食之"，是说应注意饮食卫生。至于外伤，则需在生活、工作中注意安全，留心防范。

第二节　既病防变

未病先防，是最理想的预防措施。但如果疾病已经发生，就

However, once a disease appears, it should be diagnosed and treated as early as possible so as to arrest its progress. According to the Chapter "Grand Discussion on the Concept of *Yin* and *Yang* Reflected by Various Natural and Life Phenomena" (Chapter 5) in *Plain Questions*: "The pathogenic factors seem to come as quickly as a storm does. A good doctor treats a disease caused by pathogenic factors as soon as they attack the body surface." This suggests that exopathic diseases should be cured at its initial stage in order to check its progression.

Apparently, different diseases vary greatly in their progressive patterns. For instance, the miscellaneous diseases caused by internal injury often transform according to the patterns of encroachment and violation of the five elements. Having known the features of a disease, the doctor should figure out as the first thing in the process of treatment which passgae or viscera the pathological change will approach so as to take appropriate preventive measures against its progress. The book of *Synopsis of Precriptions of the Golden Chamber* says "Doctors with preventive treatment reinforce the spleen when they find out pathogenic change in the liver, for they know the latter will certainly affect the former." When doctors deal with the pathological changes of the liver, they usually make an additional remedy to strengthen the spleen and stomach at the same time, from which the theoretical basis of the traditional Chinese remedy of liver diseases originates.

应争取早期诊断、早期治疗，以防止疾病的发展与传变。如《素问·阴阳应象大论》说："邪风之至，疾如风雨。故善治者治皮毛，其次治肌肤……。"说明对外感病应治愈于初期阶段，以防止其传变。

当然，不同的疾病有其不同的传变规律。如内伤杂病，多依五行相乘、相侮的规律传变。掌握了这一点，治疗时就应首先弄清病邪下步将传入哪一脏腑，以便采取相应的防治措施，从而制止疾病的传变。如《金匮要略》说："夫治未病者，见肝之病，知肝传脾，当先实脾。"故中医在治疗肝病时，常加健脾和胃之品，其理论根据，即源于此。

Chapter Four

TREATMENT

Section 1

Principles of Treatment

This refers to the principles in treatment of a disease, which differ greatly from therapeutic methods. Curative principles indicate the general principle guiding therapeutic methods while the methods are the specific treating techniques and subordinate to the general principle. The principles of treatment in TCM consist of the following aspects:

1. Searching for the Primary Cause of a Disease in Treatment

Contrasted with *"biao"*, *"ben"* means something fundamental or essential, just like the root of a tree. Searching for the primary cause of a disease in treatment is to seek the fundamental cause of a disease so as to make a proper remedy. This is one of the basic principles of diagnosis and treatment of TCM on overall analysis of symptoms and signs, the cause, nature and location of the illness and the patient's physical condition according to the theory of traditional Chinese medicine. In practice, however, the two aspects must be applied correctly, namely, "the routine treatment and the treatment contrary to the routine" and "treatment of *biao* (expectant treatment) and *ben* (causal treatment)".

第 四 章

治 疗

第一节 治 则

所谓治则，即治疗疾病的法则。治则与治法不同。治则是用

以指导治法的原则，而治法则是从属于治则的具体治疗方法。中

医所说的治则，主要包括以下几个方面：

1. 治病求本

"本"与"标"相对而言，有根本、本质之意，犹如树的根。治

病求本，就是要找出疾病的根本原因，确定恰当的治疗方法。这

是辨证论治的一个基本原则。但在具体应用时，必须正确掌握

"正治与反治"、"治标与治本"两种方法。

1) Routine Treatment and Treatment Contrary to Routine

(1) Routine Treatment

This refers to a routine remedy opposite to the nature of a syndrome, which can also be called "reversed remedy." Routine treatment can be applied to any syndrome whose clinical manifestations are in accordance with the nature of a disease, namely, a cold syndrome will show cold symptoms, a heat syndrome the heat symptoms, a deficiency syndrome the deficiency symptoms and an excess syndrome the excess symptoms. The remedies, however, are to treat the cold syndrome with hot-natured drugs, the heat syndrome with cold or cool-natured drugs, the deficiency syndrome with tonifying method and the excess syndrome with the method of purgation. Routine treatment is one of the most commonly used therapeutic methods in clinical practice.

(2) Treatment Contrary to the Routine

It indicates adopting a remedy according to the false symptoms of a disease, which is also called "yielding method". It is applied to those syndromes whose manifestation and nature are contrary to each other, i.e., cold syndrome with pseudo-heat symptom, heat syndrome with pseudo-cold symptoms, and deficiency in reality with pseudo-excess symptoms. Yet the nature of this method is still to treat a disease by searching for its primary causes and solving its substantial problem. The specific uses of the "yelding treatment" are as follows.

Using medicine of warm nature to treat pseudo-heat: this is to treat cold syndrome with pseudo-heat symptoms with medicines of hot nature. A typical example is written in the book *Treatise on Febrile Diseases*: "*Shaoyin* disease has the symptoms and signs as diarrhea with undigested food in the stool, interior cold but exterior heat, deadly cold limbs, deep faint pulse, preference to coldness and flushed complexion— The disease can be cured with *Tongmaisini* Decoction made up

1）正治与反治

（1）正治　所谓正治，是指逆其证候性质而治的一种常规治疗方法，又称逆治。正治法适用于疾病的表现与本质相一致的病证，即寒证现寒象，热证现热象，虚证现虚象，实证现实象。治疗则寒者热之，热者寒之，虚者补之，实者泻之。正治法是临床上最常用的一种治疗方法。

（2）反治　是顺从疾病假象而治的一种治疗方法，又称从治。适用于疾病的表现与本质相反的病证，即真寒假热、真热假寒、真实假虚、真虚假实证。但究其本质，仍是针对疾病的根本原因而治，即治病求本。其具体用法如下：

热因热用　即用热性药物治疗真寒假热证。如《伤寒论》"少阴病，下利清谷，里寒外热，手足厥逆，脉微欲绝，身反不恶寒，其人面色赤……通脉四逆汤（炙甘草 6 克，附子 9 克，干姜 9～12

of 6 grams of stir-fried licorice root, 9 grams of prepared aco-
nite root and 9 to 12 grams of dried ginger."

Using medicine of cold nature to treat the syndrome of
pseudo-cold. This is to treat the heat syndrome with pseudo-
cold symptoms with drugs of cool or cold nature. An instance
lies in the treatment of the syndrome of cold limbs due to excess
of heat, manifested as interior accumulation of heat and deadly
cold limbs, with White Tiger Decoction, composed of 18 grams of
anemarrhena rhizome, 30 grams of gypsum, 6 grams of licorice
root and 6 grams of polished round-grained nonglutinous rice.

Using tonification to treat obstructive disease. This is
to treat the excess syndrome with pseudo-deficiency due to the
obstruction caused by deficiency with tonics. For instance,
abdominal distention due to hypofunction of the spleen can
be cured with drugs invigorating the spleen with the result
of the strenthening of the functional activities of the spleen-*qi* and
spontaneous subsiding of adbominal distention.

Using purgatives to treat diarrhea and the like. This is
to treat syndromes of excess type with pseudo-deficiency
symptoms manifested as diarrhea and the like with purgatives
instead of astringent. Instances can be found in using respectively drugs promoting digestion to treat diarrhea due to indigestion, drugs promoting blood circulation and removing
blood stasis to treat metrorrhagia and metrostaxis, drugs with
heat-clearing and fire-purging functions to treat fecal impaction
due to heat with watery discharge, and drugs removing heat
by diuresis to treat frequent, quick and painful micturition
due to damp-heat in the urinary bladder.

Besides, another way "the Corrigent Method" was also
included in the method of "treatment contrary to the routine"
in books written by the predecessors. In fact, "the Corrigent
Method" is different from "treatment contrary to the routine",
and aims at anti-emesis by modifying the action of the principal
ingredients. It is actually the specific way of making up a

克)主之"，就是热因热用的范例。

寒因寒用　即用寒性药物治疗真热假寒证。如用白虎汤（知

母18克，石膏30克，甘草 6 克，粳米 6 克）治疗热伏于里、四肢厥

逆的热厥证，即为例证。

塞因塞用　即用补益药治疗因虚而滞的真虚假实证。如用健

脾方药治疗脾虚腹胀，使脾气健运，腹胀自消。

通因通用　即用通利药物治疗具有通泄症状的真实假虚证。

如用消食导积方药治疗食积泄泻，用活血化瘀方药治疗瘀血崩漏，

用清热泻下法治疗热结旁流，用清热利尿方法治疗膀胱湿热所致

的尿频、尿急、尿痛等，皆为例证。

另外，还有一种"反佐"法，在前人著作中亦常把它列为"反

治"范围。其实，反佐法乃制方、服药的具体方法，即在温热剂中

prescription and of administration. That is to add accordingly small dosage of cool-natured drugs to warm-natured prescription, or to take warm-natured drugs when the decoction becomes cold; to add accordingly small dosage of warm-natured drugs to cold-natured prescrip.ions or to take cold-natured medicine when the decoction is warm.

2) Treatment of *Biao* and *Ben*

"*Biao*" and "*ben*" are opposite to each other in concept and can be applied in many aspects. For instance, between the vital-*qi* and pathogen, the former is "*ben*" (i.e. fundamental) while the latter "*biao*" (i.e. incidental); between the cause and the symptom of a disease, the former is "*ben*" while the latter is "*biao*", and the same is true of the relations between primary disease and secondary disease, interior disease and exterior disease. In treatment of the fundamental and incidental diseases, generally speaking, one must follow the principle that treatment must aim at the root cause of a disease. But, appropriate measures should be taken in consideration of the urgency and severity of the fundamental and the incidental when treatment is carried out.

(1) To Treat the Incidental under Urgent Situation

Acute incidental disease must be given urgent treatment aimed at symptoms since delayed treatment of them will endanger the patient's life or affect the result of treatment of the fundamental of the disease. For instance, patients with massive hemorrhage of any cause should be treated with emergency measures to arrest bleeding, which means to cure "*biao*" first and "*ben*" thereafter.

(2) To Treat the Fundamental When the Condition of the Disease Permits

Causal treatment in chronic condition is to try one's best to find out the root cause of a disease for treatment when the case is relatively mild. For instance, in the case of hemiparalysis due to deficiency of *qi* with blood stasis, the deficiency of

酌加少量寒凉药，或温热剂用冷服法；在寒凉剂中，酌加少量温热药，或寒凉剂用热服法。其目的都是为了防止服药格柜而引起呕吐，与反治法不同。

2）治标与治本

标本是一个相对的概念，其含义是多方面的。如就正气与邪气而言，正气为本，邪气为标；就病因与症状而言，病因为本，症状为标；就先病与后病而言，先病为本，后病为标；就表病与里病而言，里病为本，表病为标等。标本治法的临床应用，一般是"治病必求于本"，但应根据标本的缓急轻重，采用相应的治法。

（1）急则治标　当标病甚急，如不及时治疗，将危及患者的生命或影响本病的治疗时，应采取紧急措施先治其标。如大出血病人，无论属于何种出血，均应采取应急措施，先止血以治标，待血止后再治本。

（2）缓则治本　即在病情较缓和的情况下，应尽可能找出疾病的根本原因进行治疗。如气虚血瘀所致的偏瘫，气虚血瘀为本，

qi with blood stasis is fundamental while hemiparalysis is incidental, and treatment should be stressed on invigorating *qi*, promoting blood circulation and removing blood stasis by application of Decoction Invigorating *Yang* for Recuperation, made up of 120 grams of astragalus root, 6 grams of Chinese angelica root, 4.5 grams of red peony root, 3 grams of earthworm, 3 grams of chuanxiong rhizome, 3 grams of peach kernels and 3 grams of safflowers.

(3) To Treat both the Incidental and the Fundamental at the Same Time

It used to be believed that only when both the incidental and the fundamental of a disease were acute could they be treated at the same time. As a matter of fact, treating these two simultaneously turns out to be one of the most frequently used, most effective and safest methods. It may well be concluded that the majority of syndromes observed clinically need such treatment. An instance lies in the treatment of the common cold due to deficiency of *qi*. If only the exterior syndrome is relieved, *qi* will be harmed even more; if only *qi* is invigorated, pathogens will linger. The best therapy is to treat these two aspects at the same time; to treat *"ben"* by invigorating *qi* and *"biao"* by relieving the exterior syndrome.

2. Strengthening the Body Resistance and Eliminating Pathogenic Factors

1) Strengthening the Body Resistance

This is to strengthen the vital-*qi* and the resistance of the human body as well as its self-repairing ability to remove pathogenic factors and recover the health with proper curative measures, such as traditional Chinese drugs, acupuncture and moxibustion, and some other therapies in combination with proper diet, physical exercises and Chinese *qigong*, etc. This therapeutic method can be applied to any kind of deficiency syndrome dominated by the deficiency of the vital-*qi* without

偏瘫为标。治疗可采用益气、活血、化瘀的补阳还五汤（生黄芪120克，当归尾6克，赤芍4.5克，地龙3克，川芎3克，桃仁3克，红花3克），以治其本。

（3）标本同治　过去一般认为，只有到标本俱急时，才标本同治。实际上，标本同治是最常用、最有效，也是最安全的一种治法。可以认为，临床所见的大多数病症，都需标本同治。如气虚感冒，若单纯解表，则更伤其气；单纯益气，反而恋邪。最好的治疗方法就是标本同治，益气以治本，解表以治标。

2. 扶正祛邪

1)扶正

所谓扶正，即运用具有扶助正气作用的中药，或针灸、推拿等其他疗法，并配合饮食调养、体育锻炼、气功等辅助措施，以扶助正气，增强机体的抗邪能力和自然修复能力，祛除邪气，恢

exuberance of the invading pathogens. Corresponding measures should be adopted in accordance with the specific characteristics of the disease. Instances can be found in invigoration *qi* for deficiency of *qi*, enriching blood for lack of blood and doing both for insufficiency of the two: the same is true of deficiency of *yin* or *yang* or both. All these are the specific approaches of the principle of strengthening the body resistance.

2) **Eliminating Pathogenic Factors**

This is to remove pathogenic factors with traditional Chinese drugs or some other therapies to restore the vital-*qi* and cure a disease. It is applicable to syndromes dominated by pathogens with undiminished vital-*qi*. Corresponding measures should be taken in consideration of the particular kinds and features of pathogens as well as the sites they invade. For instance, exterior wind-cold syndrome should be treated by dispelling cold to relieve exterior syndrome; lingering of toxicant substance and phlegm in the chest and stomach should be treated with emetic therapy; coproma and pathogenic heat lingering in the intestines should be treated by removing heat by catharsis; indigestion should be dealt with by promoting digestion; obstruction of blood stasis should be removed by promoting blood circulation; and interior excess of toxic heat should be cured by clearing away heat and toxic materials. All these are the specific approaches of the principle of eliminating pathogenic factors.

3) **Strengthening the Body Resistance in Combination with Eliminating Pathogenic Factors**

These two aspects supplement each other. Strengthening the body resistance helps the elimination of pathogenic factors and vice versa. Clinically, they work hand in hand. However, attention has to be paid to make sure of their appropriate positions in application according to the variations of the cases.

(1) Eliminating Pathogenic Factors before Strenthening the Body Resistance

复健康。扶正适用于各种正气虚为主，而邪气也不盛的虚证。应用时，可根据其具体病情而采用相应的治疗方法。如气虚者补气，血虚者补血，气血两虚者气血双补，阴虚者补阴，阳虚者补阳，阴阳两虚者阴阳双补等，都是扶正法则的具体应用。

2）祛邪

所谓祛邪，即运用中药或其他疗法，祛除病邪，使邪去正复，疾病痊愈。祛邪适用于邪实为主，而正气未衰的实证。应用时，可根据病邪的具体类别、性质及其在人体的部位，采用相应的治疗方法。如风寒在表，应解表散寒；痰涎、毒物停滞胸脘，宜用吐法；燥屎与热邪留滞在肠，可通便泻热；食积胃肠，当消食导滞；瘀血阻滞，应活血化瘀；热毒内盛，即清热解毒等，都是祛邪法则的具体应用。

3）扶正与祛邪的结合运用

扶正与祛邪是相辅相成的两个方面，扶正有助于祛邪，祛邪有益于扶正，故临床多结合运用。但在具体应用时，应根据不同病情，有主有次，有先有后，或同时并用。

（1）先祛邪而后扶正　适用于邪盛正虚，而以邪盛为主，急

This method is applicable to those syndromes in which pathogenic factors are excessive while the vital-qi is deficient under the domination of excessive pathogens which have to be removed quickly; though the vital-qi is deficient, it may well be competent in resistance, under which circumstances, to assist the vital-qi may reversely promote the development of pathogenic factors. For instance, metrorrhagia and metrostaxis due to blood stasis should be treated by promoting blood circulation and removing blood stasis to arrest bleeding before enriching blood, the bleeding can not be arrested without removing the stasis.

    (2) Strengthening the Body Resistance before Eliminating Pathogenic Factors

This method is applicable to syndromes of deficiency vital-qi with excess pathogenic factors under the domination of vital-qi deficiency. Under this circumstance, removing pathogenic factors will lead to the impairment of the vital-qi. For instance, at the late stage of cancer, the vital-qi is greatly deficient, the persistent using of anti-cancer drugs will accelerate the failure in the function of organism. Hence, it is essential to replenish enough vital-qi, and then to eliminate pathogenic factors with anti-cancer drugs.

    (3) Combination of Strengthening the Body Resistance with Eliminating Pathogenic Factors

This method can be applied to syndromes of deficient vital-qi with excessive pathogenic factors. It can not only strengthen body resistance with pathogenic factors repelled but also eliminate pathogenic factors without hurting the vital-qi. So, it becomes one of the therapeutic methods most frequently adopted in clinical practice. However, attention has to be paid to make clear of the primary or secondary role the two aspects respectively play. Strengthening the vital-qi is primary while eliminating pathogenic factors is only secondary if deficiency of vital-qi is dominant and vice versa if pathogenic

待祛邪；正气虽虚，尚可耐攻；若兼以扶正，反会助邪的病证。

如瘀血所致的崩漏证，因瘀血不去，则出血不止，故应先活血化

瘀，待瘀去血止后补血。

（2）先扶正后祛邪　适用于正虚邪实，而以正虚为主，正气

太虚，不耐攻伐，若兼以祛邪，反更伤正气的病证。如癌证晚期，

正气大衰，若一味地使用抗癌药物，反会加快机体的衰竭。所以，

治疗时应先扶正，使正气恢复到能够耐受攻伐时，再用抗癌药以

祛邪。

（3）扶正与祛邪并用　适用于正虚邪实证，而且两者同时兼

用，则扶正不留邪，祛邪而不伤正，临床上最为常用。但在具体

factors are dominant.

3. Regulation of *Yin* and *Yang*

The imbalance of *yin* and *yang* turns out to be the fundamental pathogenesis of many diseases. Therefore, regulating *yin* and *yang* so as to restore the relative balance of them and keep *yin* and *yang* in a harmonious state becomes one of the basic principles of clinical treatment.

1) **Removing the Excess**

That is to treat the interior cold or heat of excess type due to the excess of either *yin* or *yang* by way of excess removal. For instance, the interior cold syndrome of excess type due to hyperactivity of *yin* is treated in way of dispelling pathogenic cold with drugs warm in nature; the heat syndrome of excess type due to hyperactivity of *yang* is treated by clearing away the excess of *yang*.

An excess of *yin* can lead to impairment in *yang*, and vice versa. So, in treatment of the interior cold syndrome of excess type with *yang* deficiency, the strengthening of *yang* has to be taken into account, while in treatment of heat syndrome of excess type with deficiency, consideration should be given to nourish *yin*.

2) **Invigorating the Deficiency**

This means dealing with *yin* deficiency syndrome, *yang* deficiency syndrome or the deficiency of both *yin* and *yang* by invigorating either the deficient *yang* or *yin*. For instance, fever of deficiency type due to deficiency of *yin* is treated by nourishing *yin* to check *yang* while the cold of deficiency type due to deficiency of *yang* by invigorating *yang* to hold back *yin*.

According to the theory of "interdependence of *yin* and *yang*" held by TCM, it is essential to add certain *yang* tonic drugs to the prescriptions for nourishing *yin* when treating the fever of deficiency type due to deficiency of *yin*, namely, "to nourish

应用时，还应分清二者的主次。正虚为主者，以扶正为主，兼顾祛邪；邪实为主者，祛邪为主，兼顾扶正。

3. 调整阴阳

阴阳失调是许多疾病的基本病机。因此，调整阴阳，补偏救弊，恢复阴阳的相对平衡，促成阴平阳秘，是临床治疗的根本法则之一。

1）损其偏盛

损其偏盛，是指对阴或阳偏盛所引起的实寒证、实热证，应采用"损其有余"的方法进行治疗。如对阴盛则寒的实寒证，应温散阴寒；对阳盛则热的实热证，则应清泄阳热。

由于阴盛则阳病，阳盛则阴病，因而在治疗时对实寒证兼阳虚的，应兼顾扶阳；对实热证兼阴虚的，宜兼顾益阴。

2）补其偏衰

补其偏衰，乃指对阴或阳偏衰所引起的阴虚证、阳虚证或阴阳两虚证，应采用"补其不足"的治疗方法进行治疗。如对阴虚所致的虚热证，应滋阴敛阳；阳虚所致的虚寒证，宜补阳消阴。

根据中医"阴阳互根"的理论，治疗阴虚证时，可在滋阴剂中

the *yin* by tonifying *yang*." And to add some *yin* tonic drugs to the prescritions for tonifying *yang* when deficiency of *yang* syndrome is treated, namely, "to tonify *yang* by nourishing *yin*."

Yin and *yang* are general principles of the differentiation of syndromes in TCM. The imbalance of them can explain pathological changes of every kind of disease. Hence, broadly speaking, such remedies as relieving exterior syndrome and purgating interior syndrome, sending up the lucid *yang* and lowering the turbid *qi* and adjusting the viscera, blood and *qi*, and *ying* and *wei* can all be attributed to the terminology of "regulating *yin* and *yang*."

4. Treatment in accordance with Seasonal Conditions, Local Conditions and the Physique of an Individual

This means taking appropriate approaches to treatment according to the various situations—seasons, regions as well as the patient's constitution, sex and age.

1) Treatment in accordance with Seasonal Conditions

The climatic variations have certain effect on both physiology and pathology of the human body, therefore, they should be taken into consideration when a prescription is made. For instance, in spring and summer, as the weather turns warmer and warmer, the *yang-qi* of body is sending up and the muscles and skin are in the relaxing state. For patients even with bad cold, such drastic remedy as diaphoretics of ephedra kind must be used cautiouly in case to avoid impairing *yin* by inducing too much diaphoresis. In autumn and winter, as the weather changes from cool to cold, *yin* becomes stronger increasingly and *yang* becomes weaker, meanwhile, the muscles and viscera turn to be close and *yang-qi* is astringent internally. Medicines of

酌加补阳药，即所谓"阳中求阴"，治疗阳虚证时，则可在补阳剂中酌加滋阴药，即所谓"阴中求阳"。

阴阳是辨证的总纲，各种疾病的病理变化都可用阴阳失调来概括。因此，从广义上讲，凡解表攻里，升清降浊，调整脏腑、气血、营卫等治疗方法，都属调整阴阳的范围。

4．因时、因地、因人制宜

因时、因地、因人制宜，是指治疗疾病时，应根据季节、地区，以及患者的体质、性别、年龄等不同情况，来制定适宜的治疗方法。

1）因时制宜

一年四季的气候变化，对人体的生理、病理均产生一定影响。因而在处方用药时，应考虑到这一因素。如春夏季节，气候由温渐热，阳气升发，人体腠理疏松、开泄，即使患了风寒感冒，亦应慎用麻黄类发汗峻药，以免发汗太过，耗伤气阴；秋冬

cool and cold nature such as gypsum, mirabilite and rhubarb should be used with great care with the exception to treat extremely heat syndrome in case *yang* is hurt by purgation with drugs of cold nature.

2) **Treatment in accordance with Local Conditions**
The variation of geographical conditions, to some extent, can also affect man's physiology and pathology. The principle of treatment according to local conditions means to make up a prescription in accordance with the geographical features of different areas. Taking the common cold of wind cold type as an example, drugs such as ephedra and cinnamon twig can be used in booster dose in the bitterly cold areas than in warm areas. This is what the chapter "Discecussion on Therapies in accordance with Local Conditions" in *Plain Questions* (Chapter 12) has explained:" Why can a disease be cured with different remedies ?" Dr. Qibo replied, "Geographical conditions are different."

3) **Treatment in accordance with the Physique of an Individual**
This refers to making up a remedy according to the age, sex, constitution and life style of a patient.

Old people usually get deficiency syndrome or that of both deficiency and excess since their vital essence becomes weaker. So it is preferable for them to reduce the dosage of the drugs. Invigorators are also seldom used for babies and a re duced dosage is advisable if used, for their viscera are still delicate and their *qi* and blood are not sufficient, which make them susceptible to either cold or hear, either deficiency or excess.

Different sexes have their own features in physiology and pathology. Especially for women who are physically characterized with menstruation, leucorrhea, pregnancy and delivery, precautions must be taken in administration of drugs. Drugs with such features as drastic purgation, removal of blood stasis,

季节，天气由凉渐寒，阴长阳消，人体腠理致密，阳气内敛，故除非大热之证，当慎用石膏、硝黄类寒凉攻下之品，以防寒下伤阳。

2）因地制宜

不同的地理环境，对人体的生理、病理亦有一定影响。根据不同地区的地理特点，来考虑治疗用药的原则，即为"因地制宜"。以风寒感冒为例，如在严寒地区，麻黄、桂枝的剂量可稍重，而在温热地区，则其剂量应稍轻。此即《素问·异法方宜论》所说："一病而治不同，皆愈，何也？岐伯对曰：地势使然也。"

3）因人制宜

根据病人年龄、性别、体质、生活习惯等不同特点，来考虑治疗用药的原则，叫"因人制宜"。

老年人精气衰少，患病多虚，或虚实夹杂，故药量宜酌减；小儿脏腑娇嫩，气血未充，患病后易寒易热，易虚易实，故治疗小儿病，忌用峻攻，少用补剂，药量宜轻。

男女性别不同，生理、病理特点各异，特别是妇女更有经、带、胎、产等特点，处方用药，尤当顾及。如在妊娠期，凡峻下、

and relief of obstruction should be forbidden or administered with great care during the period of pregnancy since they will hurt fetus or be poisonous.

Men vary greatly in their constitution and in the extent of cold or heat, so the same disease can be treated in different ways. For instance, when a patient with *yang* excess is treated, drugs of warm and heat nature should be used cautiously; while cautions should be taken in using medicine of cool and cold nature when a patient whith *yin* excess is treated.

The principle of treatment in accordance with seasonal conditions, local conditions as well as the conditions of the individuals fully embodies the essence of TCM—the concept of viewing the various parts of the human body as an organic whole and making diagnosis and treatment according to the differentiation of syndromes.

Section 2

Therapeutic Methods

Therapeutic methods of traditional Chinese medicine are treatments of great specificity based on the ascertained differentiation of the syndrome and the ascertained diagnosis of pathogenic factors and pathogenesis. The traditional treatments fall into eight categories which are referred to as eight therapeutic methods: diaphoresis, emesis, purgation, mediation, warming, heat-reducing, elimination and tonification,

1. Diaphoresis

Diaphoresis is a therapeutic method that treats diseases with proper diaphoretics to disperse and relieve the exterior pathogens, mainly for the exterior syndromes and also for the early stage of wind edema, skin and external diseases such as sores,

破血、通利等伤胎或有毒之药，均应禁用或慎用。

人体的体质有强弱之分，偏寒偏热之别。因 此，虽 同 患一病，处方遣药，亦有区别。如阳盛之体，慎用温热；阴盛之体，慎用寒凉等。

因时、因地、因人制宜的治疗原则，充分体现了中医的基本特点——整体观念和辨证施治。

第二节 治 法

治法，是在辨清证候，审明病因、病机之后，有针对性地采取的治疗方法。中医传统的治疗方法有汗、吐、下、和、温、清、消、补八法。

1. 汗法

汗法是通过使人体适当汗出，以解散表邪的治法。主要用于外感表证，也可用于风水、疮疡初起以及麻疹不透等。汗法有辛

carbuncle and ulcers, and measles without "adequate eruption. Diaphoresis is subdivided into two kinds: pungent-warm relief of exterior syndrome and pungent-cool relief of exterior syndrome.

1) Pungent-warm relief of exterior syndrome: relieving the exterior syndrome with drugs pungent in flavour and warm in property. This treatment is applicable to exterior wind-cold syndrome (such as heavy chills, slight fever and non-thirst). The usual recipe contains mainly drugs pungent in flavour and warm in property that relieve the exterior syndrome, mostly having the antiseptic, antiviral and diaphoretic functions.

2) Pungent-cool relief of exterior syndrome: relieving the exterior syndrome with drugs pungent in flavour and cool in property. This treatment is applicable to exterior wind-heat syndrome (such as fever, slight chills, thirst and sore throat) The usual recipe contains mainly drugs pungent in flavour and cool in property that relieve the exterior syndrome, mostly having the functions of antisepsis and abatement of fever.

Points for attention in using diaphoresis:

(1) Sweat is a part of body fluid. Too much sweating would cause the exhaustion of body fluid. Therefore, an efficient cure for many diseases as it is, diaphoresis should never be abused. Special care must be given to the appliaction of diaphoresis to patients who lack the *yin* fluid. These patients include: ① those who suffer from severe vomiting or diarrhea; ② those who suffer from open sores and deficiency of *qi* and blood; ③ those who are deficient of *yang* by nature and suffer from frequent spontaneous perspiration; ④ those who suffer from hemorrhage or tend to hemorrhage; and ⑤ cases of measles in full eruption.

(2) Diaphoresis is not appliacble when the pathogenic factors have invaded the inner body and the exterior syndromes have disappeared while the interior syndromes have emerged. It is contraindicated to patients suffering from heart failure or

温解表和辛凉解表两种。

1）辛温解表：适用于风寒表证（如恶寒重，发热轻，口不渴）。由辛味温性的解表药为主组成方剂，多具有抗菌、抗病毒及发汗等作用。

2）辛凉解表：适用于风热表证（如发热，微恶寒，口渴，咽喉肿痛）。由辛味凉性的解表药为主组成方剂，多具有抗菌、退热作用。

运用汗法的注意点：

（1）汗液是人体内津液的一部分。汗出太多，会造成津液耗伤。因此，汗法不可滥用。对于体内阴液不足者尤应慎用，如剧烈呕吐或腹泻者；疮疡已溃，气血虚弱者；素体阳虚，常自汗出者；出血或有出血倾向者；麻疹已透发者。

（2）若邪已入里，表证消失出现里证时，则不属于解表法的

extreme debility.

(3) Differences in geographical surroundings and climate should be taken into account when using drugs pungent in flavour and warm in property to relieve exterior syndrome. The dosage and kinds of drugs may vary in different cases.

2. Emesis

Emesis is a therapeutic method to expel phlegm, saliva, undigested food or toxic substances that retain in the throat, thoracic cavity or stomach, mainly for the removal of the phlegm and saliva clogging in the throat, or the stubborn phlegm retaining in the thoracic cavity, or the undigested food and toxic substances accidentally taken that still stay in the stomach.

Points for attention in using emesis:

(1) Emesis is an emergency treatment and should be avoided except in a few very urgent cases that call for immediate vomiting.

(2) As vomiting may impair the body fluid and vital-qi, emesis is seldom advised. It is advised to try as much as possible the various other usual therapeutic methods to remove phlegm and undigested food.

(3) Vomiting brings about drastic changes of the pressure inside the chest and abdomen. Therefore, emesis is contraindicated to patients with hypertension, arteriosclerosis, aneurysm, peptic ulcer, hemorrhagic tendency of pulmonary tuberculosis and to pregnant women. For those who are too weak or suffer from heart diseases, emesis should be performed with great care.

3. Purgation

Purgation is a therapeutic method that discharges through the lower orifice (anus) the undigested food, dry stool, cold accumulation, stagnant blood, phlegm and water retaining in the stomach and the intestines by clearing up the stomach and in-

应用范围。对于心力衰竭或极度虚弱的患者，应禁用。

（3）运用辛温解表药时，其剂量与药物的选择须根据地理环境和气候的不同有所区别。

2．吐法

吐法是通过涌吐，使停留在咽喉、胸膈、胃脘等部位的痰涎、宿食或毒物从口中吐出的一种治法。主要用于痰涎壅塞在咽喉，或顽痰蓄积在胸膈，或宿食停滞在胃脘者，或误食毒物尚留在胃中者。

运用吐法的注意点：

（1）吐法是一种急救措施，除在极少数病情急剧，必须迅速涌吐者外，一般不应随便使用。

（2）因为呕吐能损伤津液和正气，所以临床上尽可能用各种祛痰法或消食法来消除痰饮和食积，应用吐法者较少。

（3）呕吐时，可使胸、腹腔内部压力产生较剧烈的变化。因此，对高血压、动脉硬化、动脉瘤、溃疡病、肺结核有出血倾向以及孕妇等禁用吐法。身体极度衰弱及有心脏病者，必须慎用。

3．下法

下法是通过荡涤肠胃，泻出肠中积滞，或积水、瘀血，使宿食、燥屎、冷积、瘀血、结痰、停水等从下窍而出，以祛邪除病

testines and excreting the stercoroma, hydrops and coagulated blood there. It is applicable to constipation due to enterogastric pathogenic factors, or to syndromes caused by the domination of pathogen and vital-*qi*, such as fecal impaction due to heat with both watery discharge, stagnant phlegm and fluid retention, blood stasis and retention of water. In clinical practice it can be subdivided into purgation with drugs of cold nature, purgation with drugs of warm nature, laxation with drugs of loosening nature and purgation with hydragogue.

1) Purgation with drugs of cold nature: This is a method to attain purgation with purgative drugs bitter cold or salty cold in nature as the major drugs supported by drugs promoting the circulation of *qi*, mainly for interior heat syndromes of excess type (high fever, constipation, abdominal distention and pain), namely, *qifen* syndrome in the middle or later stage of a febrile disease. It is also applicable to the following indications: ① early stage of dysentery due to damp-heat pathogen manifested as abdominal pain and distention with tenesmus, accumulation of heat in the stomach and intestine, marked by diarrhea accompaneid with stasis of excrement; ② fire of escess type such as conjunctivities, encephalemia, pneumorrhagia and nose bleed; ③ for food or drug poisoning, this method can help clean up the poisonous substances in the stomach and intestines.

2) Purgation with durgs of warm nature: This is a method to achieve purgation with drugs pungent in flavour and warm in nature as the major drugs supported by proper purgative drugs. It has the effects of augmenting blood circulation, promoting enterogastric peristalsis and digestion. It is applicable to syndromes such as *yang* deficiency of the spleen and stomach, cold accumulation in the stomach and intestines, hypofunction of the digestive system, slowing down of the enterogastric peristalsis, abdominal distention, abdominal cold pain, constipation or even cold limbs.

3) Laxation with emollient cathartics: This is a method

的一种治疗方法。可用于邪在肠胃而致大便不通，燥屎内结或热结旁流，以及停痰留饮、瘀血积水等邪正俱实之证。临床上可分为寒下、温下、润下、逐水等。

1）寒下：是用性味苦寒或咸寒的泻下药为主，配合行气药进行泻下的方法。主要用于里热实证（高热、便秘、腹硬满痛），即热病中期或极期的气分证阶段。也可用于下列证候：①湿热痢初期，腹痛、腹胀或里急后重，以及热结胃肠，虽腹泻而燥屎不去者；②结膜炎、脑溢血、肺出血、鼻出血等属实火者；③食物或药物中毒，用本法以排除胃肠道中的有毒物质。

2）温下：是用温里药配伍泻下药进行泻下的方法，具有促进血液循环、胃肠蠕动和消化功能等作用。适用于脾胃阳虚，冷积阻于胃肠，消化系统功能减弱，胃肠蠕动减慢，出现腹胀、冷痛、大便秘结甚或手足逆冷等证候。

3）润下：是用润肠药配合行气药进行泻下的方法，具有润

to realize purgation with emollient cathartics as the major drugs supported by drugs promoting the circulation of *qi*. It has the effects of lubricating the intestinal walls and feces, resulting in promotion of purgation. It is applicable to deuteropathic and postpartum constipation, constipation due to old age and weakness, habitual constipation, and constipation of hemorrhoid sufferers.

4) Purgation with hydrogogue: This is a method to treat hydrops by cleaning up through the bowels the large quantity of water retaining within the human body with drastic hydrogogues that lead to relatively violent purgation. It is advisable for physically strong patients who suffer from hydrothorax and ascites.

Points for attention in using purgation:

(1) Purgation is mainly used to treat interior diseases or gastrointestinal disorders and constipation. If it is syndrome still with pathogens in exterior or half-exterior and half-interior, both the exterior and interior syndromes should be dealt with at the same time; if purgation is used alone in this case, it may guide pathogens from the exterior to the interior, impair the vital-*qi* and deteriorate the illness.

(2) Purgation is a comparatively drastic method to eliminate pathogenic factors. Though having quick effects, it can also impair the body fluid. Therefore, drugs should be stopped immediately once the therapeutic effect is achieved and never be overdosed. Purgation should be handled with great care when applied to patients with deficiency of vital-*qi*, those deficiency of *yin* fluid in particular, and women in pregnancy or during menstrual period.

4. Mediation

Mediation is a therapeutic method that eliminates pathogenic factors by way of mediation or regulation, and is mostly used to treat half-exterior and half-interior syndrome. It regulates the prosperity and decline of *yin* and *yang*

滑肠壁和粪便或促进泻下的作用。适用于病后、产后、年老体弱之便秘，习惯性便秘，以及痔疮患者之便秘等。

4）逐水：用峻下逐水药，通过较剧烈的泻下作用，由肠道排出体内的大量水分以治疗水肿的方法。可用于胸水、腹水而体质较好的患者。

运用下法的注意点：

（1）下法主要用于病位在里、或具有胃肠道功能障碍和大便秘结的病人。如邪尚在表或邪在半表半里，则须表里同治；若单纯使用下法，会引邪入里，损伤正气，使病情恶化。

（2）下法是一种较为剧烈的攻邪方法，收效虽迅速，但会损伤津液。因此，在取得治疗效果后，便须停药，不宜过量。对正气虚弱，特别是阴液不足者，以及妇女怀孕期、月经期，都应慎用。

4．和法

和法是通过和解或调和的作用以祛除病邪的一种治法，主要用于治疗邪在半表半里的证候。通过调整人体阴阳的偏盛偏衰，

and thus further regulates the somatic functions under new conditions, consequently building up the patient's resistance to diseases, eliminating the pathogens and helping recover the patient's bealth. It is applicable to the derangement of visceral *qi* and blood, or to the simultaneous occurrence of cold, heat-dampness pathogens, or to intermingled asthenic and sthenic syndromes. In clinical practice mediation functions generally in the following four aspects: relieving symptoms in *shaoyang* disease; regulating the functional relation of the liver and the spleen; soothing the liver and relieving symptoms in the stomach; and regulating the functional relation of the stomach and the intestines.

5. Warming

Warming is a therapeutic method that warms the middle-*jiao*, dispel pathogenic cold and helps recover *yang*, removes obstruction in the channels and collaterals, and regulates the blood vessels by getting rid of the cold, recuperating the depleted *yang* and activating the channels and collaterals. It is applicable to diseases in the viscera and in the channels and collaterals due to pathogenic cold.

1) Warming the middle-*jiao* to dispel cold: Also referred to as warming the interior to dispel cold, this is mainly for interior cold syndromes due to the insufficiency of the spleen-*yang* and stomach-*yang*. The cold syndrome results from the hypofunction of the human body, especially the hypofunction of the alimentary system, which weakens the normal digestion and absorption, lowers energy metabolism and causes insufficient heat production and gives rise to cold syndrome. Warming the middle-*jiao* to dispel cold aims at warming the spleen and stomach, replenishing heat indirectly by promoting and strengthening the digestive function of the gastrointestinal tract so as to make up for the deficiency of energy.

2) Warming *yang* to treat collapse (depletion of *yang*):

使身体机能得到协调，从而增强抗病能力，祛除病邪，恢复健康。

亦可用于脏腑气血不和，或寒热错杂，或虚实互见的病证。和法在

临床上的运用，一般可分为四类：即和解少阳、调和肝脾、疏肝

和胃、调和肠胃等。

5. 温法

温法是通过温中、祛寒、回阳、通络等作用，祛除寒邪，恢复阳

气，疏通经络，调和血脉。适用于脏腑经络因寒邪致病的一种治法。

1）温中散寒：又称温里祛寒。主要应用于脾胃阳虚所致的

里寒证。由于人体功能衰弱，特别是消化系统功能减弱，不能正

常地消化吸收，使能量代谢降低，热量不足而产生寒证。温中散

寒，是以温脾胃为主，通过促进和加强胃肠道的消化吸收功能间

接地补充热量，改善人体能量不足的状态。

2）温阳救脱：也称回阳救逆，为疾病发展到循环衰竭时的

This is an emergency treatment used when the disease reaches the stage of circulatory failure.

3) Warming the channels to expel pathogenic cold: This is mainly applied to arthralgia-syndromes such as blockage in the channels and collaterals due to pathogenic cold, stagnation of *qi* and blood, arthralgia and difficulty in getting about. It has the functions of relieving pain and improving blood circulation.

Points for attention in using warming:

(1) Warming is inadvisable for heat syndromes, interior heat syndrome due to deficiency of *yin*, heat syndrome with pseudo-cold symptoms as well as hemorrhagic symptoms such as hematemesis and hematochecia due to heat syndromes.

(2) Certain drastic hot-natured drugs should be used with great caution on pregnant women.

6. Heat-reducing

Heat-reducing is a therapeutic method that removes pathogenic heat and fire by clearing away heat and purging fire. It is applicable to interior heat syndromes. It has the functions of antisepsis, relieving inflammation and reducing fever. It is applicable to interior heat syndromes, chiefly heat syndromes of excess type (such as the middle or climax phase of febrile diseases, suppurative inflammation), and also to certain heat syndromes of deficiency type.

1) Clearing pathogenic heat from the *qi* system: This is the usual heat-clearing method. It is applicable to indications of febrile diseases in the metaphase with heat in the *qi* system.

2) Clearing pathogenic heat from the *ying* system and from the blood: This is mainly applicable to febrile diseases in the later stage when the pathogenic heat has entered the *ying* system and the blood.

3) Clearing away heat and removing toxic substances:

一种急救措施。

3）温经散寒：多用于寒邪阻滞经络，气血凝滞不通，关节疼痛，活动不便的痹证。具有镇痛、改善血液循环等作用。

运用温法的注意点：

（1）热证、阴虚内热证、真热假寒证以及热证引起的吐血、便血等出血证，均不宜使用。

（2）某些大热药孕妇慎用。

6．清法

清法是通过清热泻火以清除火热之邪，用于治疗里热证的一种治法，具有抗菌、消炎、退热等作用。主要适用于实热证（热病中期或极期，化脓性炎症等），也可用于一部分虚热证。

1）清气分热：即一般所称的清热法，适用于热病中期热在气分的证候。

2）清营凉血：主要适用于热病极期热入营血或血分的证候。

3）清热解毒：是应用清热泻火或清热解毒类药物清泻脏腑

This is a method to clear away pathogenic fire and toxin in the viscera by using heat-clearing and fire-purging drugs or heat-clearing and detoxifying drugs. In clinical practice it is usually applied to treat bacterial infections, especially purulent inflammation due to gram-positive bacteria. It has the functions of antisepsis and reducing fever.

4) Clearing away heat of deficiency type: This is applicable to fever due to deficiency of *yin* or persistent low fever (mostly caused by physical debility, bacteriotoxin and its metabolic products affecting the vegetative nervous system and the temperature-regulating centre).

Points for attention in using heat-clearing:

(1) Heat-clearing is mainly used to treat interior heat syndromes. It should be contraindicted to cold syndromes and cold syndromes of deficiency type. It can never be used to treat cold syndromes with pseudo-heat symptoms.

(2) Most of the heat-clearing drugs are of cold or cool nature. An overdose may impair the function of the spleen and stomach and give rise to symptoms like anorexia. Therefore, administration of such drugs should not last long unless necessary indeed.

(3) For heat syndromes of excess type with damp symptoms, dampness should also be resolved by using aromatic drugs or removed by diuresis as a supporting therapy. If the heat is so excessive as to consume the body fluid, the method of nourishing *yin* and promoting the production of the body fluid should also be employed as a supporting therapy. For patients suffering from constipation, purgation is advised as a supporting therapy.

7. Elimination

Elimination is a therapeutic method that gradually eliminates the tangible lumps formed by the accumulation and stagnation of *qi*, blood, phlegm, retained food, water, worm and

火、毒之邪的方法。临床常用于细菌性感染，尤其是革兰氏阳性菌引起的化脓性炎症。具有抗菌、退热作用。

4）清虚热：适用于阴虚发热，或长期低热不退证（多因身体衰弱，细菌毒素及其代谢产物影响植物神经系统和体温调节中枢所致）。

运用清法的注意点：

（1）清法主要用于里热证，应禁用于寒证、虚寒证，更不可误用于真寒假热证。

（2）清热药物性味多寒凉，如使用过量，可损伤脾胃功能，出现食欲不振等证候。因此，如非病情确实需要，不宜久用。

（3）实热证挟湿者，宜配合化湿、利湿；热盛伤津者，宜配合养阴生津；如大便秘结，宜配合泻下。

7．消法

消法是通过消食导滞和消坚散结作用，使气、血、痰、食、

the like by promoting digestion and removing stagnancy as well as resolving masses and dissolving lumps. It includes: regulating the flow of *qi*, promoting blood circulation, removing dampness by diuresis, promoting digestion, removing phlegm and eliminating sores and carbuncles.

1) Regulating the flow of *qi*: This is a therapy that normalizes the flow of *qi* by regulating the functional activities of *qi* in the body, mainly for syndromes due to the stagnation of *qi* in the spleen, stomach, lung and liver. The therapy includes promoting the circulation of *qi*, elevating the collapsed *yang* and lowering the adverse flow of *qi*.

(1) Promoting the circulation of *qi*: This has the functions of soothing the liver, relieving spasm and pain, regulating the functions of the stomach and intestine, and arresting vomiting by using stomachics. It is mainly applicable to syndromes due to the stagnation of *qi* in the liver, speen and lung.

(2) Sending down abnormally ascending *qi*: Also referred to as lowering the adverse flow of *qi*, this is a therapy that lowers the upward adverse flow of *qi*. It has the functions of arresting vomiting, preventing hiccup and relieving asthma as well as tranquilizing the mind. It is mainly used for syndromes of reversed flow of *qi* due to the functional disorders of *qi* of the lung, the stomach and the liver.

(3) Elevating the collapsed *yang*: This is a therapy that re-elevates the descending *yang-qi*. It is applicable to diarrhea, anorexia, prolapse of rectum, prolapse of uterus and gastroptosia resulting from *qi* collapse due to deficiency of *qi*.

2) Promoting blood circulation: This is also referred to as promoting blood circulation to remove blood stasis. It has the functions of activating blood circulation and removing obstruction in the channels and vessels, removing blood stasis, promoting blood flow, regulating the smooth muscles of the various systems and organs of the human body, and relieving the spasm

水、虫等积聚而成的有形之结渐消缓散的一种治法。包括理气、活血、利湿、消食、祛痰以及消散疮疡等。

1）理气：为调整体内气机，使之恢复正常运行的治法。主要适用于脾、胃、肺、肝等气机阻滞所引起的病证。包括行气、升陷（或升阳）、降逆等法。

（1）行气：具有疏肝、解痉止痛、调整胃肠功能、健胃止呕等作用。主要适用于肝、脾、胃气机阻滞所引起的病证。

（2）降气：也称降逆法。是使向上冲逆之气重行下降的治法，具有止呕、止呃逆、止气喘、镇静等作用。主要适用于肺、胃、肝等功能障碍所引起的气逆证候。

（3）升陷：也称升阳法。是使下陷的阳气重行上升的治法。适用于气虚下陷之腹泻、食欲不振、脱肛、子宫下垂、胃下垂等。

2）活血：也称活血祛瘀法。具有活血通脉，消散瘀血，促进血行，能对人体各系统器官平滑肌进行调整，解除痉挛，从而

of the smooth muscle, thus promoting the circulation of blood and the functions of the viscera. In clinical practice it is mostly applied to treat emmeniopathy, chronic inflammation, angio-cardiopathy (such as thrombosis, vasopasm, arteriosclerosis and angina pectoris), fractures, soft tissue injuries and hepato-splenomegaly.

3) Removing dampness by diuresis: This is a therapy by using diuretics to remove pathogenic dampness. Its main function is diuresis. It should be applied with caution to those who are insufficient of *yin*-fluid. Its clinical application can be classified as follows:

(1) Inducing diuresis to treat stranguria: Mostly appli-cable to inflammation or calculus of urinary tract manifested as lower abdominal distension and fullness, frequent micturi-tion, urgency of urination, urodynia and dark urine.

(2) Inducing diuresis to alleviate edema: This is applied to treat hydrops (including cardiac hydrops, nephrogenic ede-ma and alimentary edema as well as ascites due to cirrhosis of liver). It eliminates the retained water within the body by diuresis.

(3) Clearing away heat and promoting diuresis: This is applicable to diseases or syndromes with damp-heat symptoms.

(4) Warming and resolving dampness: This is applicable to the cold-dampness syndromes due to the stagnation of water as a result of asthenia of the spleen and stomach or the deficiency of the kidney-*yang*.

4) Removing phlegm: This is a therapy that removes the phlegm stagnating in various parts of the body. It is mainly applied to treat diseases in the respiratory system. It is also applicable to certain diseases or syndromes in the alimentary, circulatory and nervous systems.

5) Promoting digestion and removing stagnated food: This is a therapy to remove the stagnated food by using stomachics that can promote the digestive function of the stomach and

改善血液循环与内脏功能的作用。临床上多用于治疗月经病、慢性炎症、心血管疾病(如血栓形成、血管痉挛、动脉硬化、心绞痛等)、骨折和软组织损伤以及肝脾肿大等。

3) 利湿：运用渗湿利水药使停滞的水湿由小便排出。其主要作用是利尿。阴液不足者慎用。临床应用可分为下列几种：

(1) 利水通淋：主要用于泌尿道炎症和结石，表现为下腹部胀满、尿频、尿急、尿痛、小便黄赤等证候。

(2) 利水消肿：用于治疗水肿(心性、肾性和营养不良性水肿，以及肝硬化腹水等)。主要通过利尿以排除体内潴留的水湿。

(3) 清热利湿：用于具有湿热证候的病证。

(4) 温化水湿：用于治疗脾阳或肾阳虚衰，水湿不能正常运行而停滞的寒湿证。

4) 祛痰：排除停留在体内各处痰邪的方法。主要适用于呼吸系统的病证，也常用于消化、循环、神经系统的某些病证。

5) 消食导滞：是运用具有促进胃肠消化功能的消导药以消

intestines. It is mainly applicable to dyspepsia syndromes (manifested as vomiting, belching and diarrhea).

6) Resolving sores and carbuncles: The sores and carbuncles include skin and external diseases as well as abscess of internal organs. They are removed and cured by the diagnosis and treatment based on their characteristics and their individual reactions and in accordance with the differentiation of syndromes, namely exterior and interior, *yin* and *yang*, *qi* and blood.

8. Tonification

Tonification is a therapeutic method that nourishes and invigorates the *qi*, blood, *yin* and *yang* of the human body. It is applicable to one or several of *zang* and *fu*-organs, or one of the *qi*, blood, *yin* and *yang*, or the weakness of all of them as a whole.

1) Invigorating *qi*: This generally refers to nourishing and replenishing *qi* of the spleen and lung. In clinical practice it is often applied to treat deficiency of *qi* (such as weakness, short breath and inappetence). Sometimes it is also applicable to deficiency of blood (as only when *qi* is sufficient in the spleen and heart can blood be generated there).

2) Enriching the blood: This is a therapy to treat deficiency of blood (pale lips, dim complexion, scanty and light coloured mensis).

3) Invigorating *yang*: This has the effects of regulating the function of the human body and promoting metabolism. In clinical practice it is mainly used to treat deficiency of *yang* (such as impotence and edema), endogenous cold syndromes due to deficiency of the kidney-*yang* (such as diarrhea and cold limbs) as well as cold syndromes due to deficiency of the spleen-*yang*.

4) Nourishing *yin*: This has the effects of regulating the function of the human body and promoting metabolism. The term "*yin*" actually includes essence of life, blood and body

除食滞的治法。主要适用于消化不良(呕吐、嗳腐气、腹泻)的病证。

6)消散疮痈：包括外疮和内痈的性质和个体反应的特点，按表里、阴阳、气血等辨证施治，使疮痈消散而痊愈。

8. 补法

补法是通过滋养、补益人体的气血阴阳，治疗某一脏腑或几个脏腑，或气、血、阴、阳之一，或全部虚弱的一种治法。

1)补气：一般即补脾肺二脏之气，临床常用于气虚证(如乏力、气短、食欲不佳等)。有时也用于血虚证(因为脾、肺、心等气充足才能化生血液)。

2)补血：临床上常用于血虚证(唇白、面色无华、月经量少色淡)。

3)补阳：具有调整人体功能，改善新陈代谢的作用。临床主要用于肾阳虚证(如阳萎、浮肿)，以及由于肾阳虚而引起的内寒证(腹泻、手足冷)，脾阳虚而引起的脾虚寒证。

4)补阴：主要具有调整人体功能、改善新陈代谢的作用。

fluid. So nourishing *yin* embraces nouri.hing essence of life, blood and body fluid.

Points for attention in using tonification:

(1) Attention should be paid to the function of the spleen and stomach (or the digestive system). Patients suffering from weakened digestive function (such as anorexia, gastric distress and abdominal distention) should first be given treatment to regulate the spleen and stomach. Sometimes digestants and drugs strengthening the spleen and stomach can be added to the tonics.

(2) Tonification can be used only when obvious syndromes of weakened body resistance are manifested. If the weakened body resistance is not serious while the domination of pathogen is obvious, major efforts should be made to eliminate pathogenic factors, or add tonics to drugs eliminating pathogenic factors to assist the vital-*qi* and strengthen the body's resistance to pathogenic factors.

(3) A patient can not depend on tonics alone. It is necessary to fully mobilize the subjective initiative of the patients who should take regular exercises and adjust their diet so as to build up a powerful physique against diseases.

As for complicated cases, one single therapeutic method can seldom satisfy the requirements of the treatment. In such cases, two or more therapeutic methods should be used in coordination to keep all the aspects in view.

所谓"阴"，包括精、血和津液等。补阴即包括补精、补血和补津液等。

运用补法的注意点：

（1）使用补法时，必须注意到脾胃（消化系统）的功能。对于消化功能减弱（如食欲不佳、脘闷、腹胀）的病人，应首先以调理脾胃为主，或于补益药中加健脾胃、助消化的药物。

（2）应用补法，必须有明显的正虚证候。如果正虚并不严重，邪实很明显者，仍应以祛邪为主，或于祛邪药中加入补益药，以扶助正气，增强体质，防治疾病。

（3）运用补法，不能单靠补药。应充分调动病人的主观能动性，经常锻炼，饮食有节，以提高自身的抗病能力。

对于复杂的病证，往往不是一种治法能完全符合 治 疗 需 要 的，这时就应选用两种或两种以上治法配合运用，才能全面照顾，治无遗邪。

Editor's Notes

Basic Theory of TCM (II) is the sequel of *Basic Theory of TCM* (I). It consists of four parts: "Pathogenic Factors", "Pathogenesis", "Prevention" and "Treatment".

The parts "Pathogenic Factors", "Pathogenesis" and "Prevention" are written by Zhang Enqin and Wang Min, the rest by Shi Lanhua.

The English version of "Pathogenic Factors" and Section Two of "Treatment" in this book is translated by Hu Zhaoyun, the rest by Han Yufang. All the English translation is revised by Zhang Enqin and Zhang Qingling successively; part of it by Yu Wenping, Xiao Gong, Zheng Yi, Zhang Shaohua, Qiao Mingqi and Mr. John Heater.

编 写 说 明

《中医基础理论》下册是《中医基础理论》上册的续编。其内容包括"病因"、"病机"、"预防"和"治疗"四部分。

本书"病因"、"病机"和"预防"部分由张恩勤和王敏撰写,"治疗"部分由史兰华撰写。

"病因"和"治疗"部分的第二节由胡兆云翻译,"病机"、"预防"和"治疗"部分的第一节由韩毓昉翻译。全部英文稿先后经张恩勤和张庆龄审校。部分章节曾经于文平、肖珙、郑艺、张少华、乔明琦和约翰·希特先生审校。

PUBLISHED ALONG WITH THE LIBRARY ARE:

· Rare Chinese Materia Medica
· Highly Efficacious Chinese Patent Medicines

《英汉对照实用中医文库》配套书

· 中国名贵药材
· 中国名优中成药

PUBLISHING HOUSE OF SHANGHAI UNIVERSITY OF TRADITIONAL
CHINESE MEDICING
530 Lingling Road, Shanghai, China

Basic Theory of TCM (II) in A Practical English-Chinese Library of TCM
Editor-in-Chief Dr. Zhang Enqin

ISBN 7-81010-105-6 / R.104

Printed in Shanghai No. 3 Printing Works.

英汉对照实用中医文库

中医基础理论(下册)

主编　张恩勤

上海中医药大学出版社出版发行

(上海零陵路530号　邮政编码200032)

新华书店上海发行所经销

上海市印刷三厂印刷

开本 850×1168　1/32　印张 4.375　插页 6　字数 110 千字

1990 年 7 月第 2 版　　1997 年 2 月第 7 次印刷

印数: 14 001—17 500

ISBN 7-81010-105-6/R.104

定价: 7.90元